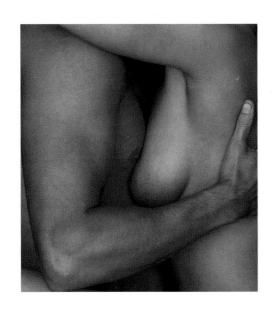

supersex

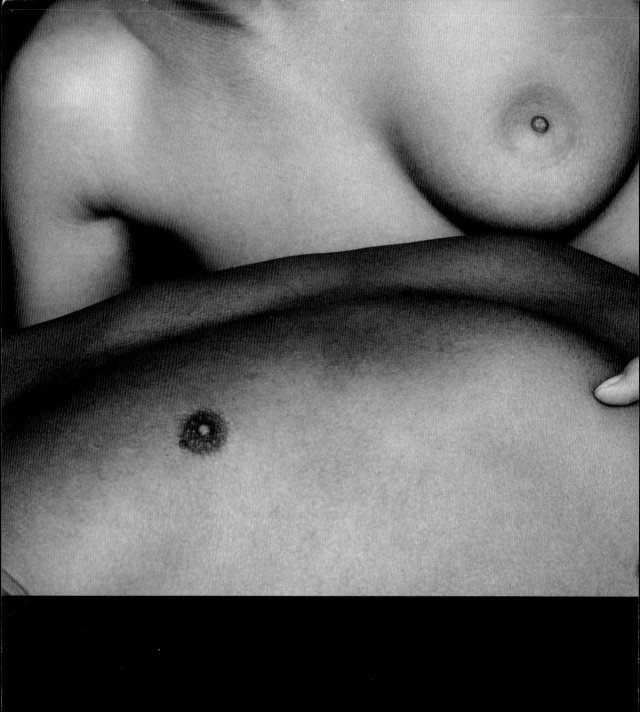

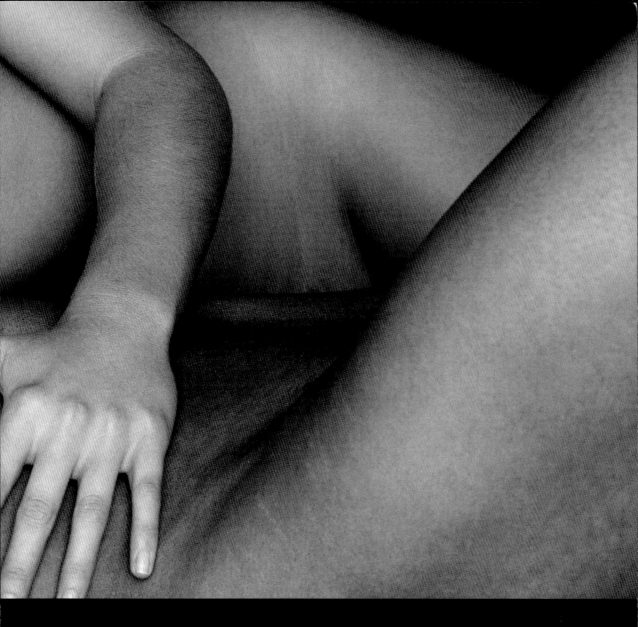

supersex

tracey cox

photography by john davis

DK Publishing

LONDON, NEW YORK, MUNICH, MELBOURNE, AND DELHI

Category Publisher
Corinne Roberts
Design
XAB Design
Managing Art Editor
Mabel Chan
Managing Editor
Stephanie Farrow
Senior Editor
Peter Jones
US Editor
Margaret Parrish
DTP Designer
Karen Constanti
Production Controller
Bethan Blase
Production Manager
Lauren Britton
Jacket Editor
Jane Oliver-Jedrzejak

First American edition, 2002

03 04 05 10 9 8 7 6 5 4 3

Published in the United States by
DK Publishing, Inc.
375 Hudson Street
New York, New York 10014

Library of Congress Cataloging-in-Publication Data

Cox, Tracey
 Supersex/ Tracey Cox; photography by John Davis
 p. cm
Includes index.
ISBN 0-7894-8959-7 (alk. paper)
 1. Sex 2. Sexual excitement. I. Title
HQ31 .C926 2002
306.7--dc21   2002067465

Reproduced by GRB, Italy
Printed and bound by Star Standard,
Singapore.

See our complete product line at
www.dk.com

Contents

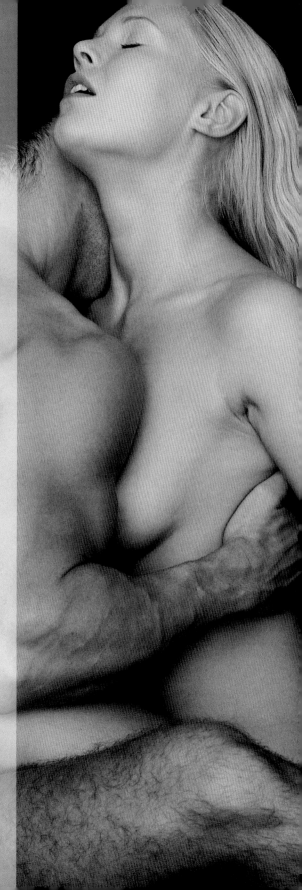

Introduction

There's sex. There's good sex. And there's supersex. I'm talking about the toe-curling, butterflies-in-the-stomach, sell-the-kids-for-more variety. The kind of sex we all want more of. The kind this book's going to help you get.

How can you learn about sex from a book? Shouldn't it all come naturally, and isn't it a little sad if you need a book to improve your love life? Ummm…no. What is sad are people who believe they are sexual mind readers, capable of mentally zoning in on someone else's desires simply by looking at, or loving, them. Nice thought. Too bad it isn't realistic. So let's get rid of that myth right here, right now: the one about love being enough. The harsh reality is, if anything, falling in love can sabotage your sex life. Why? Because you both go all gooey and get a little too considerate. Instead of flinging her across the bed and having your wicked way, you start saying things like "Oh, sorry sweetheart! Did you bang your head? Oh God, I'll never forgive myself! Are you sure you're OK?" (Surely it's a good sign if we don't notice we're practically knocking ourselves out on the headboard.) Women are just as bad once Cupid strikes. All that lascivious lip licking ("You know you want me") gets replaced by eyelash-batting ("Your mother would adore me"), as white weddings become more coveted than multiple orgasms. If it was the lip licking that won his heart in the first place, it makes sense to continue.

Don't get me wrong, I have nothing against romance or romantic sex. But I do think sex gets a bum deal in the relationship stakes, so it doesn't hurt to even up the score. There's plenty of time for the love stuff while you're in public but there's a pitiful amount of time when it's OK to have sex. So how about doing the "love you more than chocolate" thing when you're out at dinner. It's not really OK to have a quickie after the table's cleared — however tempting it is. Let lust take over during sex time. Let lust take over during the lovey-dovey parts as well, because if you really do adore each other, a degree of soppiness permeates sex anyway. Look after your sex life and the love part will look after itself.

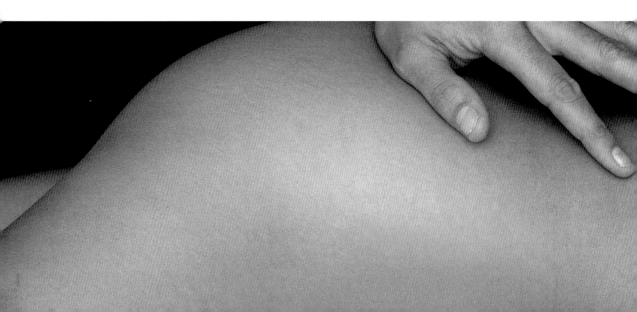

Armed with *supersex*, you'll be able to troubleshoot any problems. This book will inspire you to maintain the all-important variety you need to keep sex good long-term. *supersex* helps keep things hot because it's fun. And sex is supposed to be fun, remember? That's why parents, schoolteachers, and religious leaders keep telling teenagers not to do it. If it weren't fun, we wouldn't be tempted, would we?

Sex is supposed to be fun, remember? That's why **parents, schoolteachers,** and religious leaders keep **telling teenagers** not to do it.

supersex is sexy to look at, too. Hopefully you'll find it a fascinating read for all kinds of reasons. It's got lots of quotes, raunchy parts, and trivia that you can drag out at dinner parties when you feel like playing show-off. It's a little naughty in parts, downright dirty in others, and unashamedly slanted toward encouraging everyone to adopt a healthy if-it-feels-good-do-it attitude to sex. And while we're on the topic of free-for-alls: it doesn't matter if you're single, married – with kids or without – heterosexual, bisexual, gay, or only sleep with baboons (OK, maybe not the last one) this book's for you. It gave me great pleasure to write it. I hope it brings you great pleasure as well. In all senses of the word. Enjoy!

Tracey X

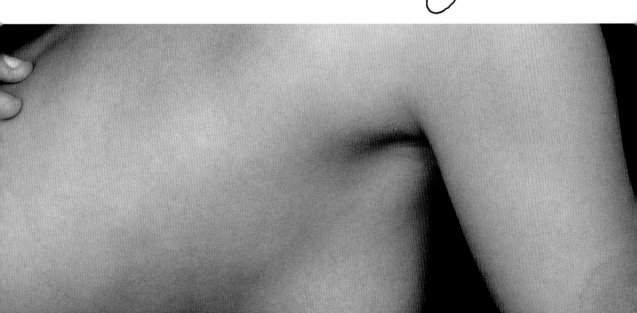

1

PLEASE

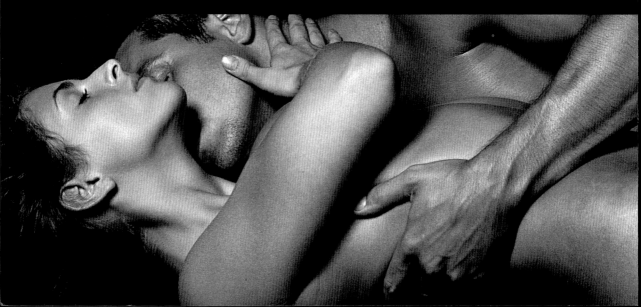

Take a magical mystery tour to find **supersecret sex spots** and **erogenous zones** you never dreamed existed. The quintessential kiss, lick, stroke, and nibble **guide to touching naked flesh**.

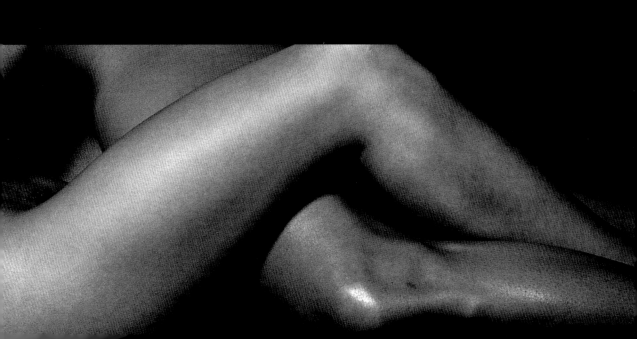

How to touch a naked man
A guided tour of his hottest sex spots

SCALP

Most people adore having their hair brushed or played with (and if he doesn't, it's usually a sign he's not in touch with himself – or you. Often it means he's uncomfortable with intimacy). A head massage isn't something he's likely to ask for (it's girly), but most men won't turn one down if it's offered and, once experienced, he'll be begging for more. It's easy to do: simply pretend you're a hairdresser who's massaging in the conditioner. Spread your fingers and nestle them in his hair, then use the pads to massage in a firm, circular motion. You should feel the entire scalp move in response.

ARMS AND UNDERARMS

Lots of women go weak at the knees at the mere sighting of a firm, veiny forearm. Others can't take their eyes (and hands) off bulging biceps. A man's arms symbolize power and virility, so it's fitting that the skin there is thick and needs a firm touch. Start by stroking your fingers up the sides of his arms, then use your whole palm once you reach the shoulders to swirl around and massage briefly, before running your palm all the way down. Make it sexier by lifting his arm and planting your mouth directly into his armpit before swirling your tongue around in large circles (yes, it's best to try it right after he's had a shower, but don't be a wimp). He's on top and you're enjoying a particularly passionate session? Bite the flesh on his shoulders – it's a novel twist on the old rake-fingers-down-back move.

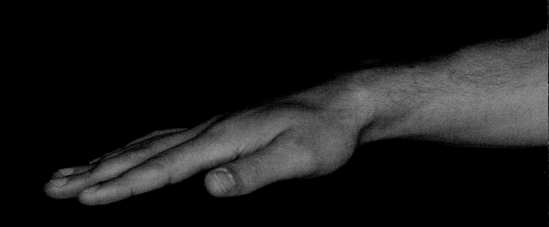

CHEST

Not only does it make the perfect pillow to snuggle up on, the chest also responds rather nicely to fingertip touches and strokes with your whole hand and tongue. Vary the pressure for better stimulation (although it's always best to work from gentle to firm, rather than the other way around). If you've got long hair, use the tips of it to tickle him. The only no-no: diving directly for the nipples. Instead, stroke everywhere but. Trail your fingertips up and down the sides of his torso (feels delicious because it's a supersensitive area), then move on to brush your entire palm across his chest, ever-so-gently, so you're skimming the hair rather than the skin. Alternate with fingertip tickling and then (and only then) tweak his nipples between thumb and third finger before licking and lightly nibbling. By the way, according to the people who study these things (and one has to question why occasionally), if you're into hairy chests, you like your men strong and masculine; if you're into the smooth or shaved look, you apparently go for the impish, boyish type.

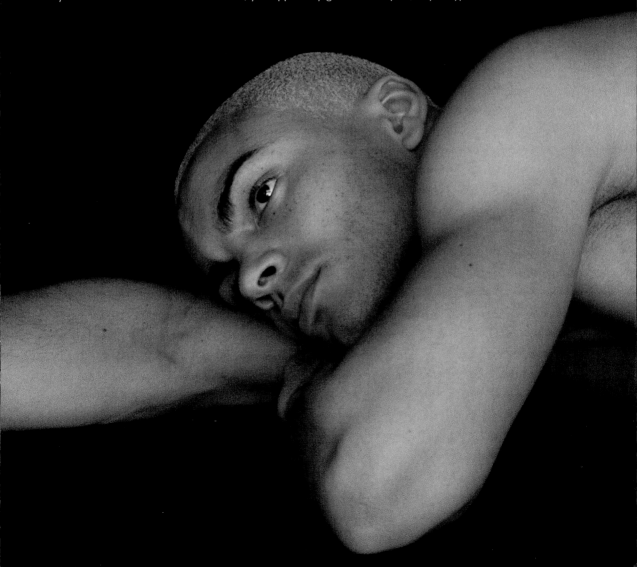

STOMACH

If running a hand over his six-pack rates up there as one of life's greatest pleasures, you'll be reassured to know that it feels good from his end too. His tummy is packed with pleasure points – particularly from his belly button down to the pubic bone. Follow that lovely trail of hair downward, stroking lightly with fingertips or tongue. Place both hands flat on his stomach and, working from side to side, move the hands in opposite directions, gliding continuously in a backward/forward motion.

BACK

Use your hair, fingertips, hands, and whatever else you like to stimulate him here. Gently stroke up the back of the neck, then move each hand off to either side, and your fingers trail down the sides of his torso before moving back up to the center of his spine. Using both hands, alternate between light tickles and a firmer motion. Finish by concentrating featherlike strokes on his lower back.

HIPS

The V-shape that's formed from his groin to his hipbones is a favorite with lots of us girls because it points to the number one body part. Which is why it's such a tease to trace it with fingers or tongue on the final run to home base. The hips are one of the most overtly erotic body parts, with jutting bones making subconscious allusions to his erection.

THIGH

The crease where his torso meets the front of the thigh is a hot zone. Use your tongue to lick upward until you hit the base of the penis where you…suddenly stop. Switch to kissing, licking, and nibbling your way up the outside of his thighs, then show mercy by doing the same on the inside.

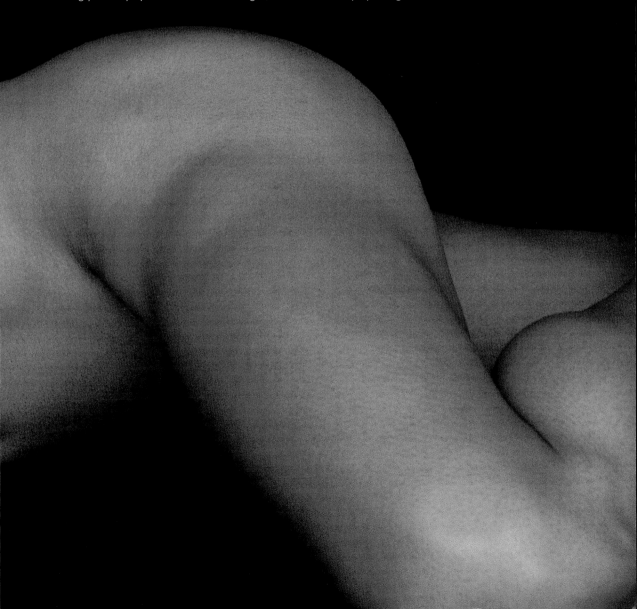

BUTTOCKS

The part where the top of his thighs meet his bottom doesn't just look good, it's extremely sensitive and a great tease zone because if you moved your fingers or tongue a fraction of an inch, you'd hit the perineum or scrotum. Use a light tickle on his buttock cheeks to start, then move into a firm, circular, kneading motion. (Don't be surprised if he jumps a little to start with, a lot of guys store tension in their bottoms and it can get very knotted up!) If you really want to make his day, lightly spank. Buttocks also make a great sexual steering wheel during intercourse: grab them and use your hands to show him how deep and fast you want him to thrust.

TESTICLES

In one survey, 99 percent of men said they loved having their testicles played with. But be gentle – the sensitivity that makes them susceptible to pleasure makes them equally vulnerable to pain. Another ouch – moving both testicles in opposite directions. Instead, hold them between your fingers and thumb and roll gently, slowly, and lightly using the pads of your fingertips. After a few minutes, put your hands underneath, so the testicles rest gently on your fingers, then using the pads, tickle them. The lighter the pressure, the more exquisite the sensation. There's also a lovely psychological kick when you touch him here because his balls are as much a sign of his masculinity as his penis.

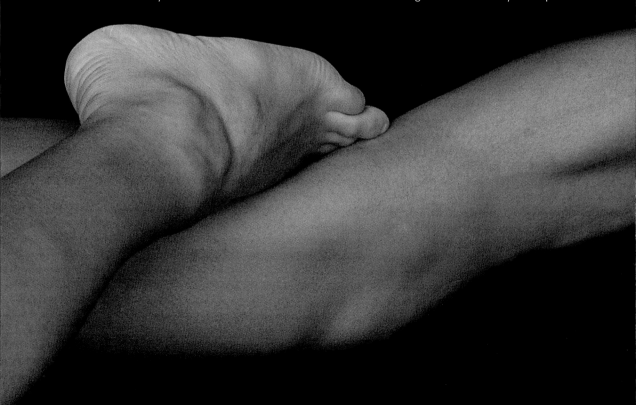

PENIS

This entire book's packed with tips on how to excite his most excitable area (see pp.76–81 for a step-by-step, hands-on guide). You can't go wrong with this basic technique though. While he's got his eyes shut, squeeze a big blob of personal lubricant into your palms, hold them together until it heats up, then make a fist and grasp the penis firmly before sliding up and down the shaft, closing your fist as you go up and over the head.

PERINEUM

It's the smooth, hairless part between his anus and scrotum which, being unbelievably rich in nerve endings, feels heavenly when massaged firmly with your first two fingers. Use a press-then-release motion close to orgasm and it often causes him to let go. Alternatively, holding the pads of the fingers firm and still can result in him experiencing the sensation of orgasm without ejaculation. Which would come in handy, wouldn't it?

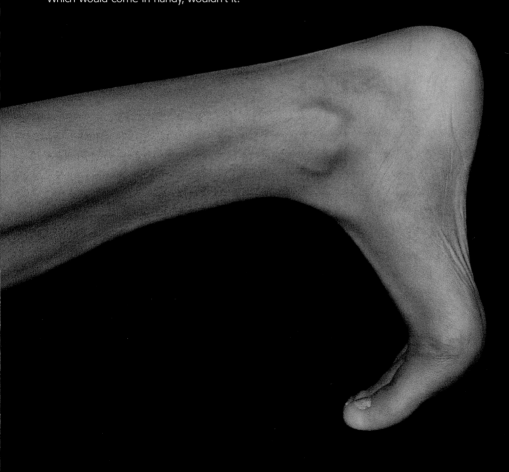

How to touch a naked woman
Know her body better than she does

FACE

Facial stroking feels exquisite and, when combined with lots of eye contact (and details of how you're about to give her so much pleasure that she's likely to lose consciousness), is a shortcut to sexual arousal and intimacy. Use a forefinger and index finger to massage the temples in a gentle circular motion, then use the pads of your fingers to stroke along every contour, particularly the jaw line and cheeks, following your fingertips with your eyes. Really look at her and let your face reflect how gorgeous hers really is.

LIPS

Besides being a literal gateway to your heaven, lips say a lot about her personality because the plumpness seems to correspond directly to how stingy or generous people are. (Translation: if she's got nicely plumped-up ones, not only will they feel better wrapped around your penis, but she's also more likely to be the generous kind and offer!) Don't waste the erotic potential of this hot zone by immediately planting a kiss smack-center with tongues flying. Instead, take time to nibble, kiss, and lick the upper and lower lip separately. Catch the upper lip between your teeth and dart your tongue lightly over it. Suck gently on the lower lip, and lick the inside of her lips as well. Make a circular trail by planting little kisses all around the edges of her mouth, and then move in for some nice, long, sexy kissing.

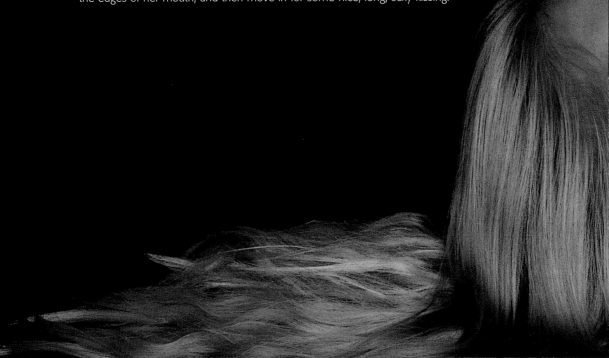

EARS

The ear is a sexy hot spot because, when you lean toward her, she's not sure if you're going to turn her on with your tongue or whisper anything-but-sweet sexual somethings. (Being the sex god you are, of course, you'll use a combination of both.) Being stimulated on the ears and earlobes sends signals straight to her internal pleasure zone. Flick and lick gently, lightly, and slowly, concentrating on the earlobes and outside area rather than inside the ear canal.

NECK

There's something incredibly sexy about being licked, nibbled, even breathed on in such a vulnerable spot. Start by brushing your lips into the hollow, where the neck meets the torso, then move into feathery kisses, alternated with tiny licks up her neck, only stopping when you hit the hairline. Start gently but when it all heats up, change the pressure of your kisses from feathery to firm, and add in a few experimental nips. If that gets a moan rather than an ouch!, she might just want you to bite!

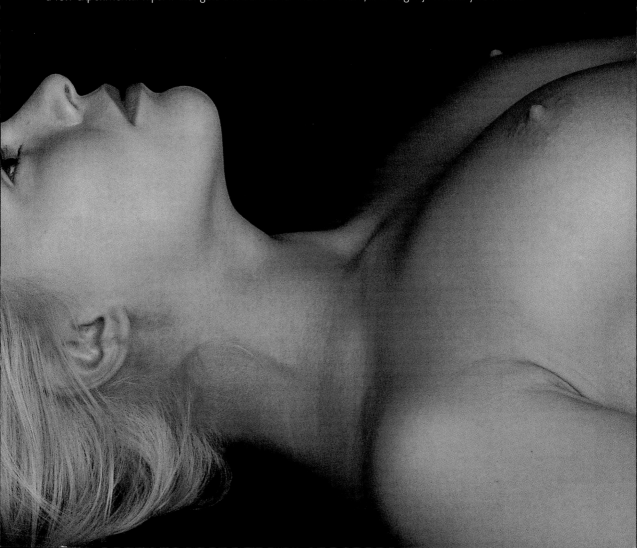

PALMS

There are 40,000 nerve endings in each palm – all just waiting to be stimulated! Use the pads of your fingers to make tiny circles, then slowly widen them. Lift her palm to your mouth and wiggle the flat of your tongue against it – the motion you use to give her oral sex. Suck each of her fingers gently while simultaneously swirling your tongue around, looking her straight in the eye all the time. It's guaranteed to make her loins liquid as she fantasizes about where the next tongue tango's going to happen.

BREASTS

The nipples and areolas (the pink skin around them) are both extremely sensitive, but also try stroking underneath, using your tongue, fingers, lips, and the tip of your erect penis as tools to tantalize. Try swirling your fingers over her breast without touching the nipples at all: a simple but highly effective tease. Combine breast-stroking with rubbing her clitoris to zap her to a place she's never been before.

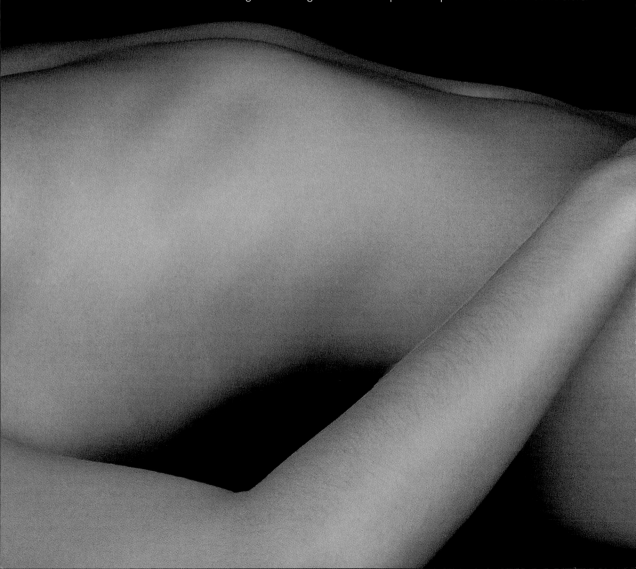

SPINE

It's the central nerve path of the whole body, so being touched on the spine is electric. Trace the entire length with your finger, retrace your steps with soft, light kisses, then flick your tongue back and forth, starting from the crease of her bottom and moving up to her neck. Now remove your mouth (if she'll let you) and use your thumbs on either side of the spine in gentle whirling movements, starting from the base of the spine and working continuously up to her neck and hairline. Also try long strokes, using the flat of the hand to run up the spine, one hand after the other, in a continuous motion.

STOMACH

Rub her lower abdomen, just above the pubic bone, as she's about to climax and see her face register an orgasm that shoots right off the raunch-Richter scale. When women experience instant lust (George Clooney comes on television – unfortunately only in one sense), we feel it in the pit of our stomachs. Have the same effect as George (try anyway) by planting your hands on her lower abdomen and slide them slowly backward and forward, moving in opposite directions across her belly.

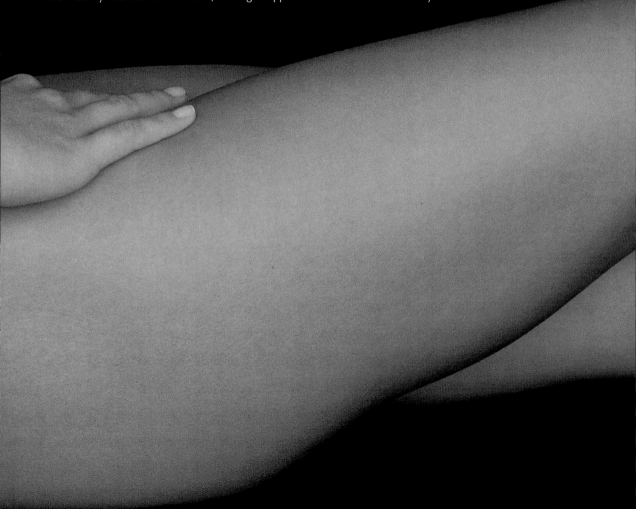

CLITORIS

Most of you know we've got one (unlike your grandad) and where to find it (unlike your dad, who still gets a little lost), but plenty of you still aren't quite sure what to do once you've gotten there. There's lots on specific techniques scattered throughout *supersex* but, as a general rule, keep all stimulation light, rhythmic, wet, and indirect (better to circle slowly around it than press it like an elevator button). As with your penis, most of the clitoris is hidden from view. The bit you see is merely the tip, underneath is the body of the clitoris, which is 1–2 inches (2–4cm), then it splits into two legs of 3–4 inches (9–11cm), which flare back into the body like a wide wishbone. With between 6,000 and 8,000 nerve endings (don't be envious, you've got the same amount on your equivalent!), it's not surprising it's where orgasms originate. The most delicious detail about this body part: it appears to have no function other than for sexual pleasure.

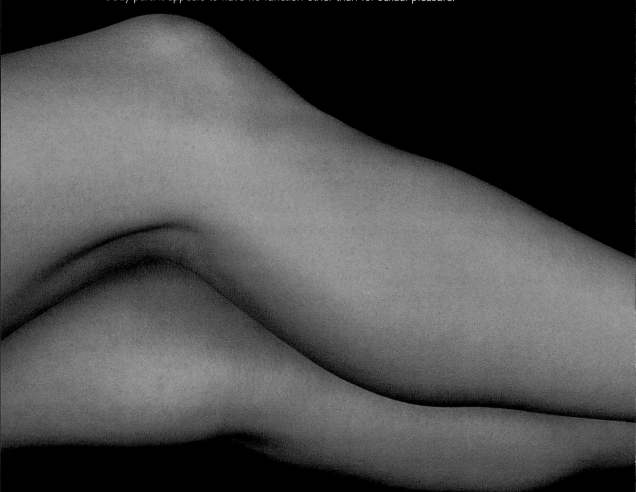

VAGINA

While your parts are out there in the open and easy to see, hers aren't. Which makes it amazing that 15 percent of women have never grabbed a mirror and had a good look around! Quite frankly, if you end up in bed with one of them, I suggest you get out of the other side immediately. If she won't take you on a personalized body tour, pointing out major attractions and possibly showing slides, you need to book your own ticket. While we all have the same parts, the exact location of them differs. The vagina is a tube about 4 inches (10cm) long. When relaxed, it contracts. When sexually aroused, it widens by about 3 inches (7.5cm) and grows 2 inches (5cm) longer to allow you to penetrate. (So those dreams – sorry, I meant fears – of "stretching" her with your penis are wishful thinking). The whole front wall of the vagina (the side nearest her belly) is wondrously sensitive. See if you can find an area that feels like the outer skin of a kiwi fruit – that's the G-spot. Insert a finger and crook it to make a beckoning motion. Initial G-spot stimulation feels awfully weird – like she's about to do the mother of all pees. Get her to grit her teeth and wait 10 seconds – the payoff is worth it.

FEET AND TOES

It's the less appealing parts of our bodies that often feel fabulous when stimulated, largely because they're not used to being explored. It's also a massive compliment, showing you find all of her sexy, not just the obvious parts. Sucking her toes sends all kinds of filthy messages to her genitals. And not just that – reflexologists say our sex drives are directly linked to a pressure point on the inside of the foot below the anklebone. Stimulate it and her by cupping her heel in the palm of your hand and using your middle finger on the pressure point. Finish with a good old-fashioned foot rub.

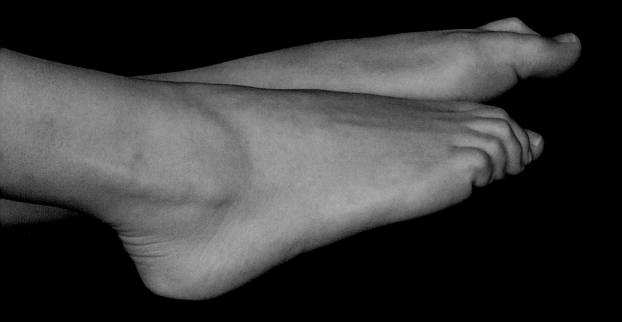

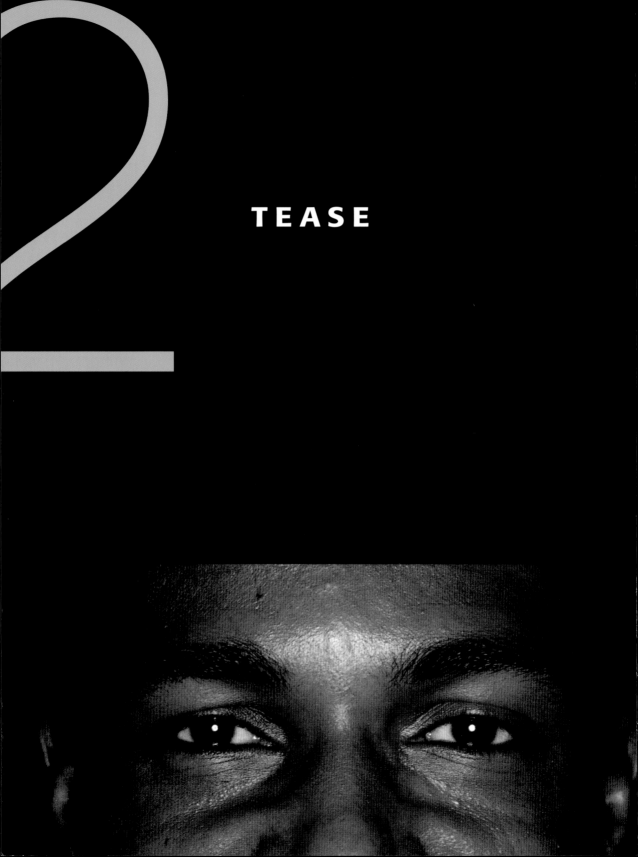

2

TEASE

Spot a great lover from 20 paces, give in to the temptation of a toy boy, and get over those first-night jitters. Plus some pretty good reasons why **making out** is a very good idea.

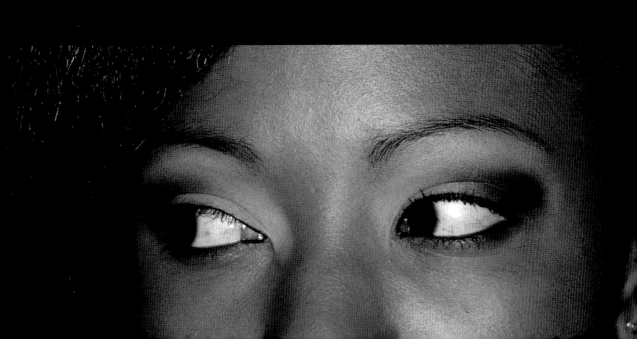

How to tell if he'd be great in bed
(without ripping his clothes off)

Ever wished you could tell what kind of lover he'd be before you jump between the sheets? Well, who says you can't judge a book by its cover! While just looking like he's dropped from heaven won't guarantee a thing, other more subtle indications are dead giveaways. Everything from the way he eats, dances, kisses, hugs, and holds your hand gives clues. How and why? It's logical if you think about it. Our clothes, mannerisms, style, appetite, and body language are all symbolic of how we are sexually – and therefore damn good indicators of how he's likely to behave in bed. Are you ready to become a sexual psychic? Here's how to figure out his sex style in seconds…

WATCH HIM EAT

The food-sex connection has been around forever and few would deny that the best lovers are hedonists: those who enjoy all the pleasures life has to offer. Never is this more evident than when someone eats. There are two types of people in the world: those who eat to live and those who live to eat. Quite frankly, I'd put my money on the guy with love handles who drools over the chocolate ads, rather than the six-pack stomach who eats one steamed chicken breast every two weeks. Why? A good appetite usually means he's got a lusty libido to match.

For signs on how he might nibble on your ear, neck or, ummm, other parts, watch the way he eats. Does he savor each mouthful of food – or simply inhale the plate? The wham-bam-thank-you man demolishes a hamburger in 10 seconds flat. The only-do-it-on-Sunday-morning-in-the-missionary-position person refuses to eat anything but steak-and-potatoes and hamburger-and-fries combos. Let's face it: if he's not into experimenting or trying exotic fare, he's hardly going to dish up the *Kama Sutra* behind closed doors, is he? Bread-and-butter taste in food = bread-and-butter sex. Even worse are the fussy, finicky types who hassle the waiter and send things back to the kitchen four times. Imagine what this guy would be like if your body's not up to snuff – let alone your sexual technique or (God forbid!) the sheets end up dirty or something! The litmus test for food, though, is if he shares. The guy who offers you a mouthful of his main course and chooses the yummiest-tastiest part for you to try is definitely a keeper. Marry the man who hand feeds you any type of chocolate dessert from his spoon.

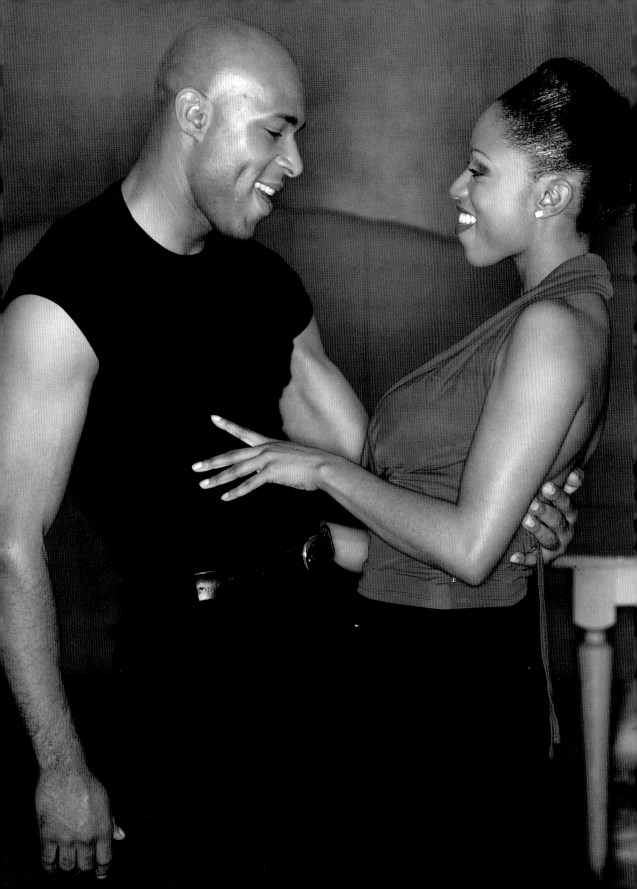

HOW DOES HE MOVE?

Someone once said that dancing is sex standing up and fully clothed. They were absolutely right – pay attention to what he does on the dancefloor and you've just had a glimpse into what he'll get up to in the bedroom. You're looking for three things: variety, rhythm, and an ability to lose himself in the music. It's for the latter reason that the self-conscious get the boot. Anyone who's doing that I'll-just-shuffle-from-one-foot-to-the-other-and-oh-dear-God-I-wish-the-floor-would-open-up-and-swallow-me thing lacks the confidence to be an inspired lover. Ditto anyone who can dance without ever moving the lower half of their body: safe bet to assume

Let's face it: if he's not **into experimenting** or **trying exotic fare**, he's hardly going to dish up the *Kama Sutra* **behind closed doors,** is he?

he's not driven by lust and would prefer to hold hands than do IT. (Romantic, sure, but do you really want a missionary man?) At the opposite end of the spectrum is the Look At Me!!!! Man. This guy's not just up on the stage but stripped to the waist, glistening with sweat, and flicking his hair around like a lap dancer…and they're playing *Mandy* by Barry Manilow. If you've got any pride at all, you'll be too embarrassed to sleep with this guy but if you do, the Look At Me!!!! Man will disappoint anyway. Sex with an overt exhibitionist is rarely satisfying. He's usually so self-absorbed, your function is simply to be a live mirror who oooh's and aaah's over how fabulous he looks and performs. Similarly, beware the guys who make jerky, hectic movements on the dancefloor. He might as well have a neon sign around his neck saying "I'm a premature ejaculator."

Instead, opt for the guy who lets loose on the dancefloor but doesn't seem to care what other people think. Someone who obviously "feels" the beat. If he can let himself go to music, then chances are that he'll be uninhibited in the bedroom as well: willing to totally immerse himself in both you and the experience. If you're crazy about oral sex, you'd cheerfully crawl over broken glass for the right tongue – ooops, I mean the right man? Then concentrate on his rhythm: a superior sense of rhythm means that he'll not only thrust well, he'll also give grrrrreat oral sex since the ability to maintain a slow, steady rhythm is essential (changing from one technique and rhythm to another rarely works).

Finally, variety: if he's only got one or two moves on the dancefloor, it usually means he's only got one or two variations in the bedroom as well. Him on top and him on top. And do I really need to point out why swivel hips *à la* Ricky Martin are an ENORMOUS plus? Oh, OK then – it's because this guy's far more likely to have perfected a circular thrusting movement, instead of the usual (boring old) up and down motion.

LISTEN TO HIM TALK

If he's talking in a monotone and changes facial expressions once an hour, you've hardly hit on Mr. Enthusiastic. Which means he'll be a bore in bed as well. The guy who's throwing his arms up in the air and nearly knocking over the waiter is full of life and passion. If he can get that worked up out of the bedroom, just think what he'll be like in it! As a general rule, the more outgoing and socially skilled he is, the more likely he is to be a good communicator in bed. The more comfortable he is with people, the better he'll connect with you sexually.

Eye contact is also important. If he can't meet your eye, he's either shy or hiding something (and it's more likely to be hide the girlfriend than hide the sausage). If he holds your gaze, rather defiantly, for long periods, chances are he'll be a bit aggressive or over-the-top intense. Ideally, he'd hold your gaze for seconds at a time, like he really does believe your eyes are the windows to your soul, but then drop them frequently so it's not uncomfortable.

Where he chooses to sit when you're out for a drink or dinner is another giveaway. If he chooses the seat facing you and the wall instead of the prime people-watching position, you're on to a winner. The more his focus is entirely on you, the more he can remain in the moment when you're alone. Never mind if Britney Spears walks in and announces he's the one she's chosen to take her virginity. He hasn't noticed a thing. He's so riveted on you – what you look like, what you're saying – nothing is going to distract him. Now imagine all this single-minded attention focused on giving you pleasure and you'll get a fair idea of what's in store for you. Exactly.

HOW'S HIS TOUCH?

I'm not talking whether he pinched your butt on your way to the restroom, but whether he's generous with his affection. Does his baby sister get a huge hug hello? Do his male friends get a firm handshake and a warm pat on the back? Or is he stiff and rigid when others dare to invade his personal space, keeping everyone at arm's length? The more comfortable he is with expressing affection, the more affectionate and loving he'll be during sex.

How close he stands dictates whether he wants to get as up close and personal as you do. If he's ready to pounce, he'll move closer. If he's too nervous to stand too close, he's going to be petrified to take it further (which means you have to make all the moves). It could also mean he's standing back in all senses. If things have progressed to the hand-holding stage, you've got another batch of clues. How he holds your hand is a significant indicator, not just of how he'll perform in bed but how he'll feel about you afterward. If he intertwines his fingers with yours, he's likely to be highly erotic: he's touching every part of your hand, expressing a desire to be connected to you physically and emotionally. This boy's not afraid of intimacy. At the opposite end is the man who does a half-hearted, fingertips-only hand hold. Words like "lukewarm lover" and "commitment-phobe" should spring to mind here, though shy and unsure are also possibilities. He opts for the standard palm-to-palm clasp? This shows affection and acceptance though it's unlikely he's going to surprise you sexually.

LET HIM HOLD YOU

If he puts both his arms around you and rests his hands on your bottom, it's a blatant invitation for sex. If he pulls your bottom in close so both your lower torsos are pressed tight, God help you if your boss/mother/ex-boyfriend is watching.

The guy who walks along holding you in a shoulder lock (elbow around the neck, arm dangling in front of you) is being friendly as well as intimate. He's a laid-back guy with a casual attitude to life – and sex. This doesn't (necessarily) mean his heart's not in it but it does mean he's interested in having a fun time, rather than a heated, heavy session.

You disappear into his big, tight bear hug? This is good news. It means he's likely to be open, loving, and not scared of involvement. If it's such a full body squeeze you can feel each other's

If he gets a little **carried away** during the **kissing session**, even better – who wants a **lukewarm lover?**

heartbeats, prepare for the roller coaster – the tighter he grips you, the more involved he wants to be. The sexiest hug of all, though, is if he wraps both arms around your shoulders and pulls you right up to him. If you're touching at the shoulders, the body naturally moves forward at the hips, turning an innocent hug into…a groan-making groin grind.

HOW'S HIS KISS?

The clincher! If it's melt material, so will the sex be. If it's awful, don't go there (and why would you want to if you're not even enjoying first base?). Think about it. If he's taken time to perfect his kissing technique, he's probably not one of those I-have-magnets-on-my-hands-and-your-breasts-are-made-of-metal men. If he refrains from shoving his tongue down your throat, he won't rush you into sex (expect foreplay galore). If he gets a little carried away during the makeout session, even better – who wants a lukewarm lover? Men who cup your face in their hands before moving in for contact are romantic souls who want to gaze lovingly at your face – or they're intense, passionate lovers who want full, reciprocal focus. Most promising sexually is someone who'll kiss with their lips and touch you somewhere else with their hands at the same time. A kiss is far more arousing and erotic if he's got you in a lip-lock and his hands start caressing your back or waist. This is the equivalent to saying, "Can I remove your clothes please? Like – NOW!" The award for The Most Promising Lover based on just a kiss, however, goes to the guy who uses a variety of kissing techniques – nips, chews, bites, and licks – and really explores all of your mouth. (If I need to point out why that's a good sign, go straight to pp.60–67. Got the picture?)

Portrait of a cheat

Using a combination of personology (that's face reading to the rest of us), university studies, scientific research, and body language signals, the experts have come up with this portrait of an unfaithful man. (Ohmigod, I'm describing your boyfriend???!! While I wouldn't dump him on the spot, you might want to remove the rose-colored glasses!)

- **He's tall** Shorter men have lower levels of testosterone, so aren't ruled by their penis and (sorry guys) aren't flirted with as much.

- **His eyes are wide apart** He's easily bored and tempted by anything in a skirt. Best bet: guys with close-set eyes. Once he's committed, he won't cheat.

- **He's got Hugh Grant hair** No wonder Hugh cut off the floppy locks: they're a dead giveaway of infidelity. Men with hair that is short at the sides and longer at the front are self-centered, self-obsessed, and least likely to worry about the effects of an affair on you.

- **He's a big drinker** Men who drink no more than the recommended weekly total (sensible drinkers rather than boozers) are 82 percent less likely to commit adultery than heavy drinkers. Don't be too smug if your boy's addicted to caffeine instead: coffee drinkers are twice as likely to be unfaithful.

- **He's a big boy** Yes, unless you're incredibly inventive, you might need to indulge in some foreplay to find out this one. But the size of a man's testicles is a scientifically proven indicator of his fidelity. The bigger they are, the more sperm he produces and the more of a slave he is to his libido.

- **Looking suspiciously at your partner?** Relax if his face is oval. An oval face means home and family are important to him. He's unlikely to stray unless pushed too far.

The size of a man's **testicles** is a scientifically proven **indicator of his fidelity**. The bigger they are, **the more sperm** he produces and the **more of a slave** he is to his libido.

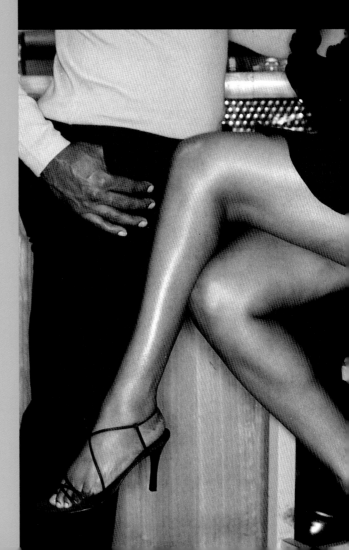

Single vs. couple sex Who's got the best deal?

Are you missing out on fabulously frivolous flingettes that leave you on a natural high if you're already sharing your bed and the remote with someone? Or do sleepy Sunday morning "spoons" count for more than you think?

SINGLE SEX

One of the sexiest, most liberating moments of my life happened when I was freshly single. It was during one of those yummy, heady times, when you're feeling free, decidedly horny, and out there after having left an excuse-me-if-I-yawn long-term relationship. I was touring with a group of male strippers, editing a magazine based on a male cabaret act. In other words, getting paid to hang around gorgeous muscly blokes and write about them. (I know – I spent many a sleepless night tossing up whether or not to take that job.) Anyway, after a few nights backstage, averting my eyes during costume changes and then not bothering, I was pretty immune to all this naked flesh. Except for Ethan.

Ethan had the body of a Greek god. As the tour went on, I found myself falling for him. Scratch that: I found myself in one hell of a lust lather. One night I also found myself four-Chardonnays tiddly. And it was just Ethan and I in the changing room after a show. I'm not being coy here, but I'm not one for sex-without-strings. But I hadn't had (good) sex in a long, long time and I knew Ethan quite well by then so he wasn't really a one-night stand, was he? He was in the middle of pulling his clothes on when there was this moment: he looked me straight in the eye and stopped getting dressed and I looked him straight in the left bicep and thought…Oh screw it! Screw being a good girl and being professional!

We moved in for what should have been a sennnnnnsational kiss, and in anticipation, angels burst into song. Then, inexplicably, they were calling my name – or someone was. And it wasn't Ethan or the angels. Turned out to be some friend of Ethan's who just happened to choose that moment to visit him backstage and who just happened to be the winner of a beauty contest *Cosmo* had run the year before and guess who was on the judging panel? She recognized me as one of the judges and I was standing there smiling at her thinking "Oh, how humiliating!" and wondering just how much she's seen, even though nothing ever really happened. Are you disappointed? Imagine how I felt!!!!!! Ironic that my sexiest moment didn't actually involve any sex whatsoever.

But that's sort of the point because single sex is all about that split second before it happens: the moment before you're about to kiss/bed the person you've been fantasizing about for weeks/months/three minutes. The reason why it's so exciting? You've never ever been together before. And that, in essence, is one (if the only) area where single sex beats couple sex hands down.

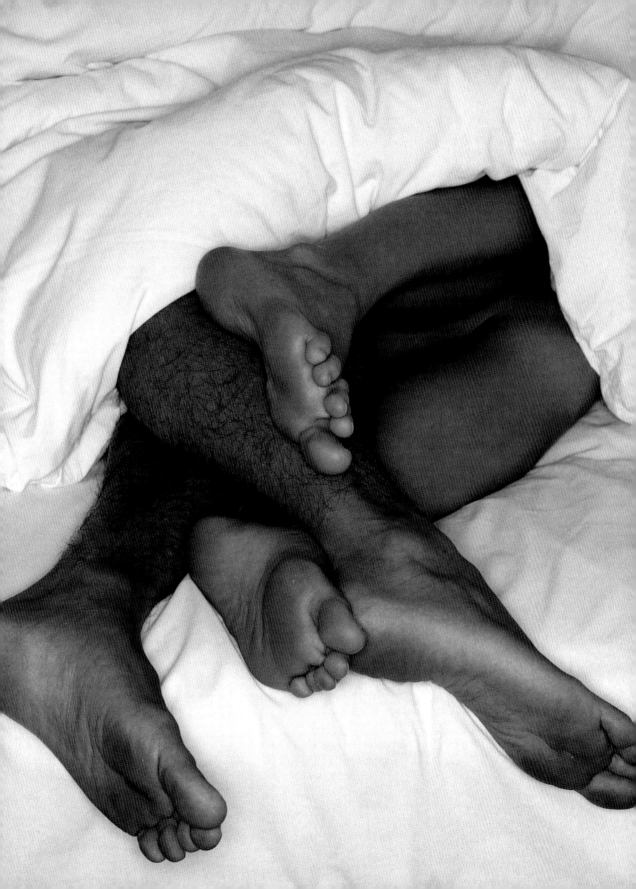

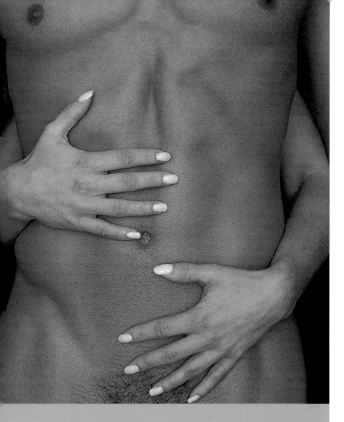

Sex with a stranger

The good: If you haven't had sex for ages, one wicked weekend can boost much more than your sexual confidence. Your pheromones – the chemicals that kick-start your libido – get a boost because you "absorb" pheromones from your partner during intercourse.

The bad: In terms of technique, it's unlikely to be great. You don't know them, they don't know you, neither of you has a clue what turns the other on, and it seems a waste of breath (pant, pant) to tell them, just for this once. Go for chemistry. The cute boy you've been talking to for four hours is relationship or friendship material, not a fling.

The ugly: Please tell me I don't need to tell you to use a condom. But even if you use one, it won't protect you against things like herpes and crabs. The emotional fallout isn't great either. Don't even think of sex with a stranger unless you know you're not going to beat yourself up about it the next day.

The main plus of single sex is the newness factor. The main drawback of couple sex is not having the newness factor. Which is, of course, why people try to cheat by having a little on the side (and end up losing it all because no one wants to have sex with someone who lies).

It's also naughty. Even if it is now OK to have one-night stands, one part of us still thinks we're not supposed to, which of course makes it infinitely more exciting. The sense of detachment can be really arousing: feel free to talk dirty, act out a fantasy, scream the roof off, because who cares if they judge you? It's not like you're auditioning to be their date for the company Christmas party.

On the downside, no-strings sex is selfish: you're both out for your own pleasure and the sex is pretty hit-or-miss. Even if it's not that bad, it can still feel pretty empty and pointless lying there with someone you don't know and don't particularly want to know. Especially if you feel like snuggling but aren't sure if it would be welcome, and you think you'd probably better not because you've got no intention of going back for seconds…and you don't want to lead them on. (Having sex to get to snuggle at the end is never a terribly good idea.)

It's not just women who feel like this, by the way. If you believe what most people tell you, all men would prefer to sow their wild oats and play the field rather than chew them contentedly in a nice, green meadow with a white picket fence. Right? Wrong. Both men and women crave relationships. It's true, men are better at separating sex from love – they've had more practice at it and are given the go-ahead to do so by society. It's also true that men generally sleep with more partners than women do (though women are catching up). Again, that's because society allows men more lovers than it does women. But that's where the differences between the sexes end. Men don't turn green and froth at the mouth if they don't get laid every day. It's the same for both sexes. Your sex drive has got a lot more to do with where you're at in your life, how you're feeling/looking, or what you're looking for, than your gender does.

COUPLE SEX

One of the sexiest, most liberating times of my life happened when I was in love. "Hang on a minute," I can hear you say, "Didn't you just say that about single sex?" Ummm, yes. But I'm allowed at least two sexy moments in my life, aren't I? This one happened with a very, very special ex, and recalling all this, the reason why I ended it suddenly escapes me. We were eight months into the relationship and at our peak. We touched each other constantly, felt frantic with need if separated for a night and swapped lots of those things-I've-never-told-anyone stories. But most exciting of all, we were great in bed together. Look up "sexually compatible" in the dictionary and you'd find our picture. We pushed each other to try stuff we normally wouldn't, but balanced that out with lots of soppy, stare-into-each-other's-eyes, loving, lazy encounters. Not to mention one HUGE dollop of chemistry; we were close to sexual nirvana. I'd been in love before. I'd had great sex before. But I'd never had so-good-your-toes-curl sex with someone I wanted to marry. Let's be honest here: how often do you find a combination of all the above elements in one person? OK, it didn't last forever, but it was still an extraordinary time in my life. Single sex might have its ups but if you've got the right partner, couple sex has it all.

Men don't **turn green and froth** at the mouth if they don't get **laid every day.**

While you can have great sex with someone you don't love, great sex with someone you do lends new meaning to the term "orgasmic." The more sex you have, the more sex you want. Orgasms are (or at least should be!) frequent and constant – you know each other so well, you know what buttons to push. Crucially, there's trust. While some are much more likely to walk on the wild side with a stranger, others find they're more open to new adventures with a partner they know and trust.

The downside of couple sex is being stuck in a bad sex cycle. If you're single and have bad sex, you walk away and try your luck elsewhere. If you're married or in a relationship, you're stuck with it. Even worse, you're forced to do what everyone dreads: work at the relationship. (Ughh!) Another harsh reality: while you'd have killed for sex-on-tap when single, once it's just a matter of turning over, it isn't half as appealing. Happily the highs far outweigh the lows – probably because couples experiment more with different lovemaking moods. In addition to the swing-off-the-chandeliers-type sex that singles have, you have sensationally soppy spoon sex, sex where you both laugh yourselves stupid, and sex where you both stop halfway through, hug fiercely, and say, "God, I love you!" Sweet!

Stripped bare!
The secrets of stripping

Is your stripping for him his ultimate fantasy? Is the Pope Catholic? I made all my male friends read the instructions that follow and asked, "If your girlfriend did this for you, would you be impressed?" "Impressed?!!" spluttered my friend Sean, "I'd be on my knees if a girl did this for me." (To propose, by the way.) I enlisted the help of an expert on this one. The gorgeous Amy Bateman is a London-based dancer, stripper, and teacher of both arts. She helped put together this idiot-proof strip routine (and yes, she does get asked out a lot).

THE TOP TITILLATING MOVES

Set the scene for seduction by e-mailing or calling your partner earlier in the day. His instructions: to buy champagne and have it on ice by the time you get home. When you're ten minutes away from the house, call again and ask him to put on your chosen CD (time it so the right song will be playing when you walk in the door), turn the lights down a little, and plonk his bottom on the sofa. Then take a deep breath and prepare to…

Walk the walk Throw open the front door (well, maybe not too violently in case he's hovering behind it) and carelessly throw your handbag in a corner. If he's not already sitting expectantly on the couch, order him there. Then simply parade about a bit, strutting your stuff. Mentally visualize a figure of eight and make your hips follow. Place one foot directly in front of the other when you walk and you'll see how easy it is! Chest out. Head up. Think proud and sassy. It's all about attitude!!!! (And OK, you're allowed one rather large gulp of champagne.)

Play with your "penis" No, I've not gone nuts. Your scarf – the modern girl's equivalent to the feather boa – is your phallic object. Treat it as you would him: sometimes rough, sometimes gentle. Run it seductively through your hands, then over your shoulders and from side to side, arching your back at the same time (stomach in, breasts out). Scarves are great props: use it as a blindfold, put it around his neck to draw him close, use it later to tie him up (but only if he's been a good boy).

Remove your jacket As an Object of Teasing the jacket comes off very, very, v-e-r-r-y-y-y slowly. With your back to him, look back over your shoulder. Unbutton the jacket, then shrug your shoulders sexily so it slides down in one motion. Remove one arm at a time but DON'T drop it! This is what separates the professional from the amateur: a real stripper will keep the jacket covering her bra and breasts. Hold the jacket over your breasts with both hands and…then turn around to face him. Remove the jacket from your breasts with one hand and drop it to the floor.

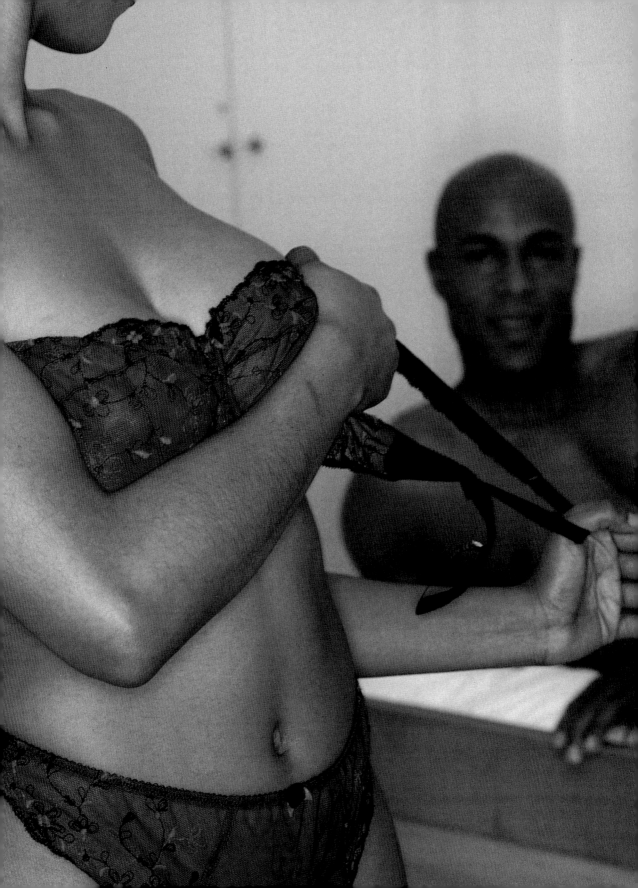

Off goes the skirt Again, with your back to him, look over your shoulder. Unzip your skirt as slowly as possible, sticking your butt out and arching your back. The skirt should be off in one quick, smooth motion. Once it's on the floor, step out of it and leave it there. A word of warning to the clumsy (like me): it's easy to get it caught around your ankles, do an ungainly dance, then topple in an undignified, humiliated heap – which is why one gulp of bubbly is good for the courage, but more is a bad idea.

And the high-heeled shoes Slip-on mules aren't optional, they're *de rigueur*. There's not really an elegant way to remove your shoes but the whole effect is instantly ruined if you're having to stop, lean over, and fiddle with straps. (I don't care how gorgeous they are or how thin they make your ankles look, you're NOT allowed to wear them!) Simply lift your leg up behind you, lean down, and use your hand to remove the shoe in as "ladylike" a way as possible.

Slide off your stockings Position yourself side-on, maintain eye contact, and put one leg up on a chair. Undo the garter belt first (obviously), then roll down the stockings using both hands, one on each side of your leg. Keep it nice and slow – the idea is, your hands are his hands. Keep rolling down until your hands are on your ankle. (Butt high in the air, of course!) Once you've slipped the stocking off your heel, remove it from your foot with finger and thumb, then use it as a prop to drape around his neck, swishing it past his nose so that he can smell the scent of your skin on the stockings.

Ping the garter belt   These don't look so hot without stockings attached, so get rid of yours right after the stockings have been removed. Simply unclip and ping them across the room with as much finesse as you can possibly muster! And hopefully without removing one of his eyes.

Braless and brazen Stripping for him is a little like unwrapping a present when the prize inside is you. Every time you peel off a piece of clothing, he's closer to seeing what's hidden inside, so draw this one out as much as possible. Face him, then shrug the straps off nice and slowly. Turn around, look over your shoulder (maintaining eye contact), and undo the bra but hold it over your breasts. Now turn to face him (a suitably wicked expression on your face) and with one arm across your chest, holding the bra in place, use your other hand to pull the bra out from beneath, nice and slowly. Drop the bra but keep one arm still covering your breasts. Then take it away, stroking your fingers across each breast as you go. Now's when you go into full stripper mode: back arched, breasts out. Play with and touch them, lifting them in both hands, kneading the nipples. Make like Demi in *Striptease*.

Next – the undies! OK, the idea is to remove your panties porn-star style, instead of yanking them down as if you're going to pee. Whatever you do, don't have your legs together for this one or you really will look like you're about to plant your bottom on the nearest toilet seat. Keep one leg in front of the other with your heel lifted. Got the stance? Get ready for the finale! Put your hands (palms facing legs) completely inside the straps at the side so you're lifting them up and away from your legs. Give him a side-on view, then slide your hands and panties down your body, keeping them lifted away from your body. As your hands move down, your body follows. Once your undies are past your knees, they should fall down to your feet. Now for the final (and hardest) part. If you thought stepping out of your skirt was hard, stepping elegantly out of a teensy-weensy, all-curled-up-like-a-rubber-band thong is a nightmare. The best advice Amy can give: take it slow and step out one foot at a time.

Take a victory lap The temptation is to rush over and hide in his. Don't. Parade around, touching and caressing your body until he can't take it anymore – and needs to take you instead.

THE TEN GOLDEN RULES

1. **Absolutely totally cannot be broken rule No. 1** You're allowed to touch him, but he's not allowed to touch you. Not with hands, mouth, tongue, or penis. Only his eyes and imagination are allowed to roam.

2. **Absolutely totally cannot be broken rule No. 2** You must maintain eye contact with him throughout the performance.

3. **Keep the lights ON** It's all about showing off your body, not hiding it. It really doesn't matter whether you'd put a supermodel to shame or make the local preacher's wife look good, sexy is all about how you *feel*. You don't need a great body to strip. All you need is confidence and attitude.

4. **Slather on stuff…** Fake tan (you'll feel more confident with some color), lip gloss (slightly smeared), blusher (around your nipples to make them look more defined), a slight slick of baby oil on your body for sheen.

5. **Plan your outfit** I've deliberately made this strip user-friendly in the sense that it assumes you've just come home from work and walked in the front door. Sure, you wouldn't normally wear stockings and garter belts to the office (top score if you do!), but there's not too much else that's different – which means you'll be far more likely to strip on impulse (and therefore actually do it, rather than just talk about it). There's only one thing Amy and I absolutely insist on outfitwise: no big underpants *à la* Bridget Jones! Obviously, a G-string (thong) suits the mood of a striptease best but it's far more important that you feel sexy in whatever underwear you choose.

6. **Don't be a neat freak** You're supposed to be throwing your clothes off with abandon. Stopping to put your skirt on a hanger, carefully folding your top, or hanging your jacket behind the door ruins the effect somewhat (don't laugh – it happens). Everything is left where you throw/drop it.

7. **Think the three T's: tempt, tantalize, tease** During the entire performance, parade around, walk up and down, flirt, flick your hair around, gyrate your body. Be his private dancer.

8. **Your hands are his hands** Touch yourself the way he wants to touch you, in places he wants to touch. Go for it. You can keep it light and innocent by touching yourself the way a virgin might. Or you can get wickedly down-and-dirty from the word go.

9. **Borrow a dancer's trick** Keep one leg in front of the other, heel lifted, whenever possible. It makes otherwise awkward poses look elegant (and your legs and body look long and lean). It's also great for photographs (check out any shot of Liz Hurley and she's invariably assumed this pose)!

10. **Choose the music to suit your mood** Yes, "Hey, Big Spender", is a tad dated, so just choose something you always end up flinging yourself around the living room to, on your wilder late nights.

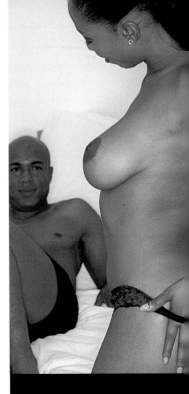

You're allowed to touch him, but **he's not allowed to touch you.** Not with hands, mouth, tongue, or penis. Only his eyes and imagination are **allowed to roam.**

Tempted by a toy boy?
Why the older woman/younger man combo makes perfect sense

It's official, by the way: age means zilch. In the past, scientists have stuck to the evolutionary theory that men prefer younger women who are likely to bear them more children. Not so. Results of a recent study show that men don't really care how old a woman is, it's what she looks like that counts. (Oh hang your heads, you shallow creatures!)

While there's an obvious downside (the good-looking really do rule the earth), the upside is you don't need to be nearly so panicky about aging as you think. In this study, a group of twenty-something men consistently chose the attractive forty-something woman over lots of younger, if plainer, women. And it wasn't just for a quickie either. Another study guaranteed to fill you with joy claims you're likely to be much better in bed even if you're just two years older than he is than the girl who's two years younger. Whether it's power, charisma, or the fact that you're a damn good lay, the older woman is a hot property. So next time you're stressing about wrinkles or arms that continue waving when you've stopped, remind yourself of six reasons that make the older woman hotter than the latest pinup…

1. OLDER WOMEN KNOW WHAT THEY'RE DOING

By the time most sexually adventurous women hit 30, they've been through more than a few lovers. And, like anything, the more experience you have at something, the better you are at it. Over the years, the older woman has dealt with penises that won't go up, down, or do both in the same amount of time it takes to say "premature ejaculator." She's had lovers who needed their left shin tickled to get turned on, those who needed instruction on just about everything, and some who've taught her a thing or two. Her younger counterpart might have breasts that point to heaven but an older woman will keep you floating on cloud nine through sheer sexual knowledge.

2. OLDER WOMEN TAKE CHARGE

She's not afraid to direct on position, pace, or foreplay – and if needs be, literally take matters into her own hands. The sight of a woman masturbating is a strong aphrodisiac for men (understatement of the millennium). She's capable of satisfying her own needs – which takes the pressure off. If he didn't make the earth move for her, he can drift peacefully off to sleep knowing she's both willing and able to cause a few rumbles of her own. Because of the age difference the older partner invariably becomes "teacher," the younger partner "pupil." While this can be restrictive out of bed, it sometimes works well

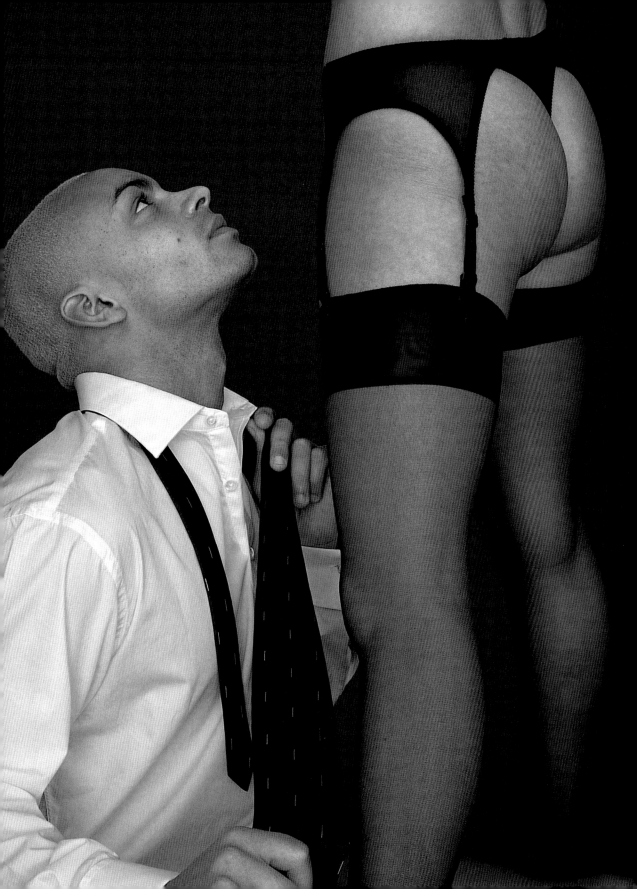

in it. Plenty of women still lie back and expect the guy to do all the work. If she takes the lead and becomes the sexual aggressor, it's an automatic penis-pumper. He's young, with flesh that's both willing and able — she's got the imagination and the guts to take him where she's already been.

It's nearly always good news if the woman takes control of a sexual relationship because women focus less on intercourse and orgasms. Sex is about giving each other pleasure, not simultaneous climaxes. Older women have also had longer to grapple with issues like "Will he think I'm easy if I suggest that?" (God no, he'll love it!), so are more open to living out the fantasies he's been harboring for years. Age also lends valuable insight into the male sex drive. If you've got a few good, long-term sexual relationships under your belt, you've figured out that men adore novelty. Give him lots of visual stimulation and new things to try and he's not going anywhere.

3. OLDER WOMEN SWALLOW

Every last drop. I know, I'm being hypocritical here because I'm the first to say swallowing isn't the be-all and end-all of giving great fellatio, but the idea of it remains the stuff of his fantasies. It scores BIG brownie points. So does good oral sex technique. An older woman knows how to give oral sex without appearing to choke herself (she's done it a hundred times more than the 19-year-old he last slept with); secondly, she's over that uugghhh-yukky-get-it-off-me sperm stage and has rightly decided that brief moment of bitterness on swallowing is worth the pleasure it gives him.

4. OLDER WOMEN TAKE THEIR TIME

It usually takes women a little longer to get warmed up than men. An older woman doesn't apologize for this, she makes the most of it, knowing a slower, longer sex session is likely to be a lot more enjoyable for both of you. He might be able to climax on cue, but a delicious buildup makes his orgasm more intense as well. An extra bonus: by letting him arouse you fully, you're reciprocating with the biggest turn-on of all — responsiveness. He really would rather have dimpled thighs that quiver than a perfectly smooth set that don't move an inch! Many men name responsiveness as an even bigger turn-on than beauty.

And while we're on the topic of looks — it's ironic, but older women worry less about their bodies than younger girls do. It's not that they don't care what they look like, they just tend to be more accepting of their bodies. The type of woman who's inclined to go out with a younger man is usually pretty attractive — she cares about keeping her body healthy and looking good because, let's face it, physical appearance is nearly always the initial attractor. Followed closely by sex appeal. If you're in your sexual prime (which usually hits post-30), your sex drive is also high (think dog in heat). Which means your sex pheromones are pumping like crazy and being picked up on a subconscious level by any man who comes (ahem) within 20 paces. If you're on the prowl, you also tend to hold your body in a rather show-off sexy manner. Stomach in, chest out, buttocks tight. Give the guy a break, he can't help but notice you!

5. OLDER WOMEN ARE ADORING

My friend Ian sums it up beautifully with this memory, which still makes him sigh 12 years later: "The best time of my life happened when I was about 20 – and I still haven't met anyone who's remotely measured up since. I was in really good shape and muscly back then and teaching diving at a resort in Fiji. Kate was about 38 and one of my clients. Her husband was too, but he spent most of the vacation doing his own thing. Kate and I went diving and ended up sitting on this secluded little beach. I peeled off my wetsuit and she started running her hands up and down my chest and arms and kissing me. For ages she just looked and felt every muscle, my skin, everything. I felt like a Greek god. I've never been so turned on in my whole life."

6. CONFIDENCE = CHARISMA

A confident lover is always in demand – no matter what she looks like. In fact, plenty of therapists say it's an older woman's sexual confidence that is at the heart of her appeal to younger men. If there's just one other piece of advice a young girl should take from an older woman it's this: you won't get what you want in bed unless you ask for it. If an older woman wants her partner to touch her breasts, she'll take his hand and put it there. Lots of younger women refuse to guide their lovers because he should "know" what to do, or fear he'll take instruction as criticism. Wrong. Most men would love a more hands-on approach.

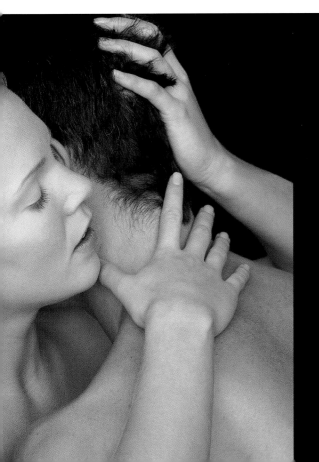

Toy boys tell all

"When I was 15, I'd find myself checking out women 5–10 years older instead of the young girls. They seemed more curvaceous, they had an air of mystery about them, they were sensual."
Simon, 22, sales representative

"You don't pick older women up, they pick you up. You make eye contact and they don't break it – and, of course they're better in bed. They're less inhibited, and willing to do a hell of a lot more."
Mike, 21, design student

"Older women aren't hanging around waiting for a man to fill their life. She has her own life already: you don't become her life, you become a part of it. You get more freedom to be your own person."
Nathan, 25, bar manager

Kissing: not just for kids
Why regular tonsil-touching sessions are a very good idea

Close your eyes, get in a time machine and cast your mind back to when you were a 14-year-old and making out under the bleachers. Whatever happened to good old petting, huh? Back then you'd spend hours locking lips. As "grown-ups" we ignore the pleasures of puckering up because it seems more adult to be aiming for multiple orgasms.

Which is a damn shame really, because a good kiss gets your knees trembling, your heart racing, and your groin aching. Some really intense kissing transports you to another world – one inhabited only by your mouth, your partner's, and the delicious sensations you're experiencing. Our mouths, tongues, and lips are a minefield of sensory apparatus: packed with nerve endings, they're remarkably responsive. Kissing also stimulates production of endorphins, the natural opiates of the body, giving you an unbeatable, and natural, high. Some people claim they're able to reach orgasm through kissing alone. Try out these techniques and you might just join the club!

THE STEP-BY-STEP GUIDE TO THE PERFECT KISS

- **Smell your breath** In one recent survey 71 percent of people rated bad breath as THE top turn-off to getting up close and personal. Garlic breath puts off one in three; smoking will stop one in four people from wanting to kiss you.
- **Kiss your palm** I'm serious. I know, it's a little like practicing by sucking on oranges like you used to when you were about 11 years old. But seriously, unless you're planning on doing it while sitting in traffic, who's going to know? Your palm is sensitive enough to pick up on the different tongue techniques and you'll get a good idea of what works and feels good and what doesn't.
- **Kiss their palm** The perfect kiss starts way before your lips lock with theirs. So start by taking their hand in yours and raise it to your mouth. Then look them straight in the eye and bury your tongue in their palm, swishing it around. Don't tense your tongue, relax it, and use the entire surface rather than just the tip.
- **Now, hold their face in your hands** This gives you ultimate control since it puts you in boss position. (Even better if you're female: it's unanimous in pretty much all sex surveys that men love take-charge kissing). Tilt your head to one side, look them deep in the eyes, then close your eyes and start moving in toward them as s-s-s-s-l-o-w-l-y as you can.

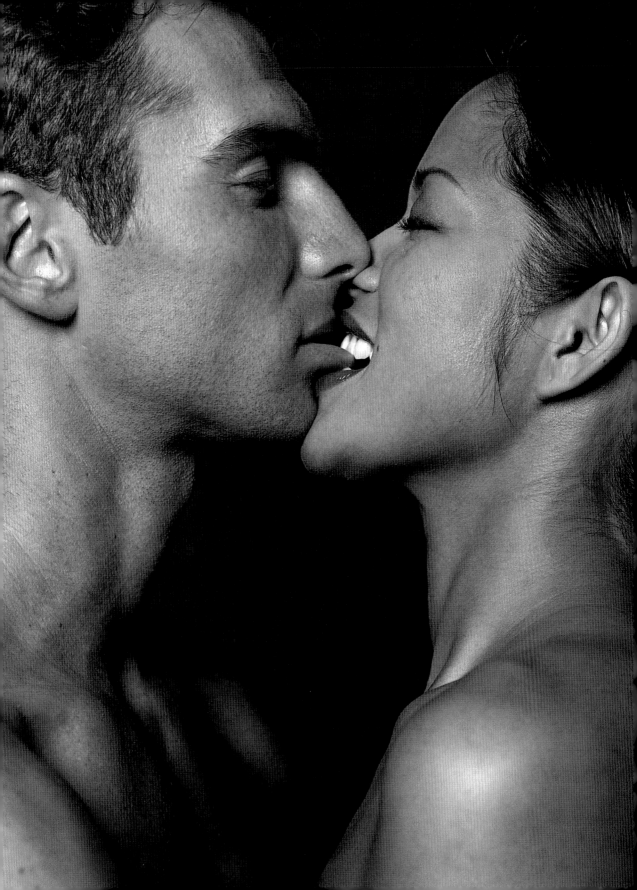

- **Start soft** Keep your lips closed (but only just, not clamped tightly together), then cover all of your partner's mouth with light, fluttery "angel" kisses until you've left your mark on every inch. Kiss in the corners, above the top lip, below the bottom lip, all around your partner's mouth.

- **Detour to the neck** Keep planting soft kisses across their face, then walk your lips down the neck until you reach the hollow. Once there, open your mouth wide and plant your lips. Make some slight suction to suck some flesh between your front teeth. Give a little nip/tug, then release. When you're aroused, endorphins are released into the bloodstream that not only create intense pleasure but block pain receptors. This explains why a mischievous nip is more likely to feel good during lovemaking – but it's still not for everyone. Another thing mouths are great for: asking questions – such as "How do you like to be kissed?"

- **Back up to the lips to nibble** Take your lover's bottom lip and trap it between your teeth. Twist it slightly then use a nip-and-nibble, suck-and-tug motion. Do the same to the top lip. Nibble in the corners, to the side, and smack in the center. The top lip is more difficult to get to so you might need to reposition yourself. Try kissing upside down. Stand behind them while they're sitting on the couch. They tilt their head back, you lean over them to kiss so your faces appear upside down to each other. According to Tantrics and Taoists, the upper lip is the sexiest part of a woman. Hindu sex books claim there's a nerve which runs directly from the upper lip to the clitoris! Enough incentive to explore this one, boys?

- **Open your mouth, lock lips, and move into a traditional kissing motion** This bread-and-butter technique basically involves pressing your lips against your partner's and moving your mouths. Think what a fish does with its lips and imitate. The easiest way to vary this kiss is through the pressure. Contrast soft, gentle kisses with harder, passionate ones as you get more excited.

- **Use your tongue** The absolute worst kissers tense their tongues until they turn into ironing boards, stick it in your mouth, and then leave it in there. Which is sooooo erotic. Not. An alternative to the sophisticated tongue-shoved-down-the-throat technique is to hold your mouths close together, lips slightly apart, and take turns letting your tongues flick across the surfaces of your lips. Try moving the tip back and forth, then imitate a figure eight. (Ever wondered how "French kissing" got its name? Credit appears to go to the Maraichins, from Brittany, France. They invented *maraichinage*: a technique of kissing "where lovers' tongues caress the inside of each other's mouths for long periods").

- **Moan** Letting out even a tiny moan/sign/groan of pleasure while your lover's mouth is on yours takes the eroticism through the roof because it creates vibration and brings another sense into focus: sound. Sound is a neglected sense in the bedroom, since most people don't make nearly enough noise!

- **Put your fingers in your partner's mouth** Pull back from kissing, lock eyes, then put one of your fingers in your own mouth to moisten it. Using your fingertips, lightly trace the outline of your partner's lips, until you've circled the whole mouth. Leaving your fingers hovering near the outside corner, lean in for a good kiss, then slide your middle finger inside the mouth, close to the corner. Use your finger to slide along the edges of your tongues and to generally explore what your mouths are doing. A good lover will lick your fingers while they're in there. It sounds weird but try it: it's highly erotic if the atmosphere is hot and heavy enough.

- **Bite – carefully** Hickies are worn with pride when you're 12. Not so when you're forced to make a presentation to a major client, with an audience of 15 staring at the purple love bite on your neck. It doesn't exactly scream "I was lying in bed worrying about this meeting last night." Besides, you can get the sensation without having to leave lasting reminders of lust. Instead of sucking away like a vacuum cleaner, take a fold of flesh between your teeth and use your lips and mouth to create slight suction and sensation. Practice on your palm and you'll instantly feel/see the difference between doing this and rhythmic sucking, which is what leaves a mark.

- **Oh all right, the tongue again** If you're really, really, REALLY turned on, even an avid stiff-tongue-hater like me admits this can work. All you do is use your tongue to imitate the longed-for thrusts of your pelvises. Or wait until you are having intercourse and make your tongue a second penetration. It's also useful to set the pace subliminally. (If you want him to thrust slower with his pelvis, thrust slower with your tongue. Speed things up by speeding up your tongue movements.)

- **How long should the perfect kiss last?** The jury's out on that one. Statistics show the average kiss lasts around three and a half minutes with only one in six of us claiming kisses of five minutes or more. Men are twice as likely to not mind if a kiss lasts less than a minute – and less likely to enjoy one that lasts five minutes or longer. (Unless it's extraordinarily sensual – which, of course, yours will be after all this training!)

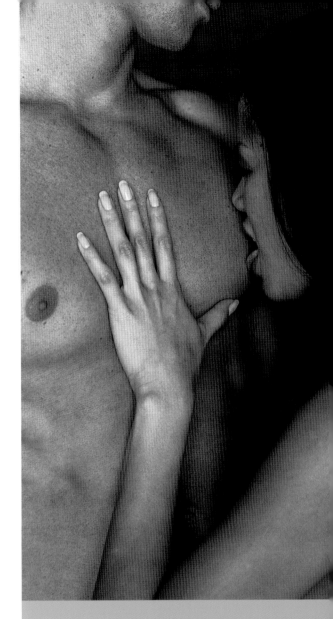

The average **French kiss** burns 12 calories **– a lot of lip-ups** for one chocolate bar, but the concept's appealing.

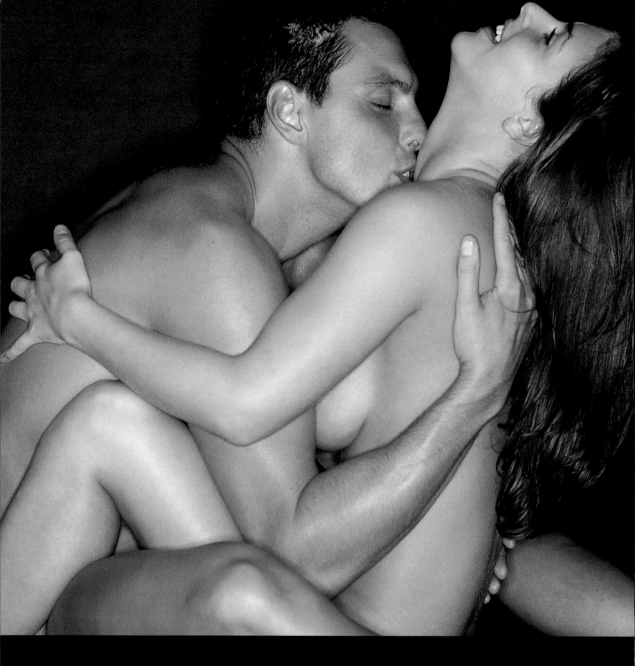

Doubly delicious: the champagne kiss

All you need is a bottle of bubbly, your partner lying on their back, and you straddling them. Take a good gulp of chilled champagne into your mouth, resist the urge to swallow. Now, lean over and kiss your partner, letting a tiny amount of champagne trickle into their mouth. Wait until they realize what you're doing and swallow, before letting a little more trickle out. The more turned on you get, the bigger the gulps. Even better if some overflows down the sides of their mouth – you've got the perfect excuse to lick it up. Only one word of caution with the champagne kiss: it's highly addictive, making it fairly easy to get sloshed. Don't forget to take turns being the giver and receiver.

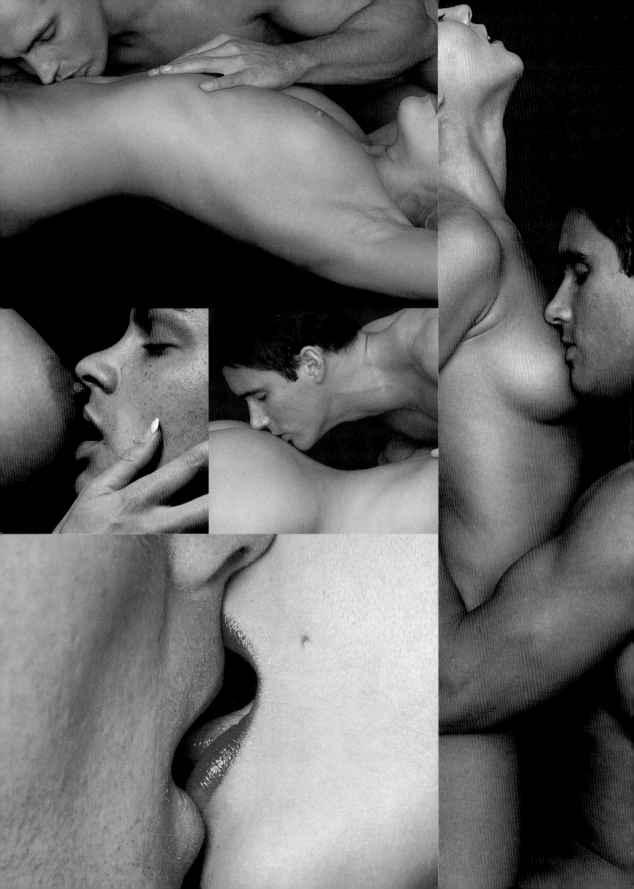

Virgin on ridiculous
Beating those this-feels-like-the-first-time-all-over-again jitters

With so many marriages ending in divorce, many of us are being rudely shoved out of cozy coupledom to land, flat on our backs, smack bang in the middle of the singles scene. Thought you'd never have to stare at a strange ceiling ever again? Yup. You're in for all that once more.

Here's more good news: if you thought it was hard the first time around, when you were soooo much younger, it's even worse baring your bod to a complete stranger when the only person to see your saggy parts (other than your partner) in the last decade has been the cat.

I know, when your last relationship fell apart, you vowed you'd never fall in lust again, let alone love. Now here you are wanting to get naked with someone – and trying to convince yourself it's no big deal. After all, it's hardly as if you're a virgin, is it? You've done "it" before. So if it's not such a big deal, why do you feel so…well, completely and utterly petrified?

Because sex with someone you like and want to build a relationship with *is* a big deal. Allowing someone to see you naked – to feel, smell, and taste your body – does make you vulnerable. And I'm not even talking about the emotional complications and dangers that intimacy implies. I'm just talking about the physical part. The part when a million weird and worrisome thoughts spill into your brain faster than the champagne you're gulping down in a vain attempt to stop them. Will my body be good enough? How will I compare to their ex? Will this be a turn-off? Will they notice the scar on my back? Do I have a zit on my butt? Is it any wonder your heart's going pitter-patter-thud-thud? Fortunately, anxiety isn't the only thing that's making your heart race. After all, we are talking about sex with new flesh here. Which is enough to raise even Aunt Martha from her sexual deathbed in about one second flat. So, on D- (Do It) Day, you find yourself seesawing between feeling as nervous as hell and as excited as can be.

How does all this translate to the bedroom? Not terribly well, quite frankly – particularly for him, because penises tend to follow their masters. Meanwhile, as a woman you're lying there torn between wanting to show off all you've learned after years of reading *Cosmo* and not wanting to seem too experienced. What to do? Keep reading.

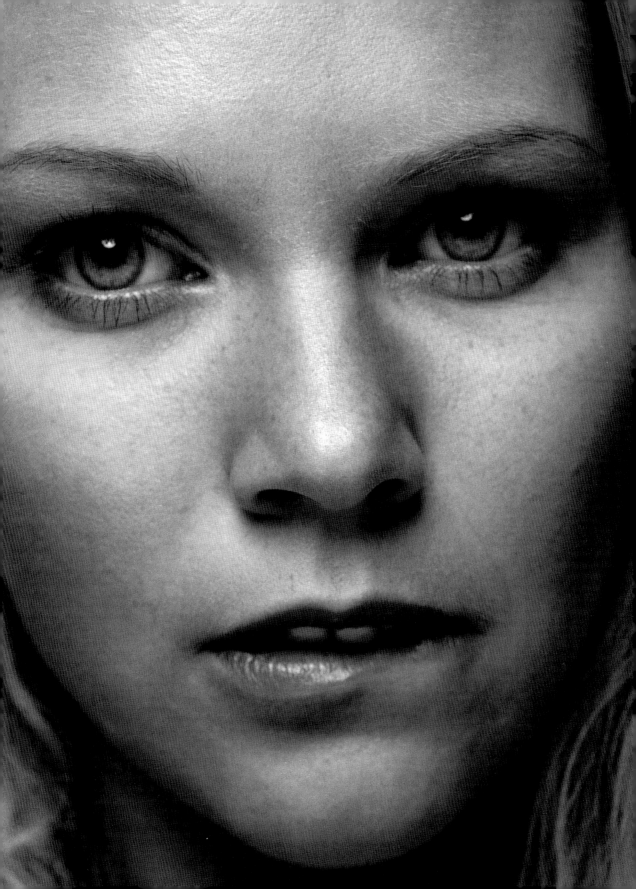

What he's thinking

Oh my God, she's actually going to let me do it. Right! You down there. Yes, I'm talking to you. OhpleaseGod, pleaseGod, pleaseGod behave. We've talked about this, remember? Don't even think about doing that hang-your-head-and-shuffle-your-feet-thing! You're meant to burst through my boxers saying, "Hi, about time we met" in a silky James Bond voice. Now, wake up!!! This is bad. Really bad. Worse than I thought. I thought you'd introduce yourself, wine, dine, do your bit, and be back home surfing channels and eating pretzels, before I even had the chance to say "Oops! Sorry!" Come on. Let's at least try for some kind of coordinated effort. Think, think. Think about her. Better still LOOK at her. She's just gorgeous!… OhthankyouGod, you're working. Fannnnntasstic. Right. What to do now? OK, calm down. I calm down but get her excited, that's it. Kissing done. Breasts done. Lots of licking. Girls like licking. Going well. Erection happening. Erection t-h-r-o-b-b-i-n-g. Oh help. Better stop licking…but she'll hate me. Keep going. No. Oh shit, stop NOW! Oh no, if looks could kill – that was one hell of a glare she gave me just then. Sorry but I…OK. Right. Do it. Just do it. Onward and upward. Kiss her first though. Concentrate. Control. Control. Control. God – she's so hot, so sexy – and – she's putting it in there already and I'm not mentally psyched up to – ohmiiiGODDDD it's just so wonderful in here. Oh hell! Have to stop. Have to keep going for at least half an hour. Think big underpants. Think Mrs. Cartwright in 4b. Count backward from 500. 499, 498. Is she? Does that groan mean she's about to…ohhhhhhhhhhhhhthankkkkkkkkkkyyyyyy yyyyyyyyyooooooooouuuuuuuuu…Damn, damn, damn, damn. I've blown it.

COUNTDOWN TO A FABULOUS FIRST TIME: ON YOUR MARK…

- **Think about contraception and safer sex** Thinking someone's awfully sweet/drop-dead gorgeous does not mean you won't wake up with an awfully painful not-so-gorgeous blister on your whatnot.

- **Think about timing** Do it when you feel ready, not because society expects it or your friends say you should. Take your time, take it slow, get to know each other first.

- **Set the scene** Too much styling and it'll look contrived, but you can make sure there are clean, crisp sheets on the bed.

GET SET…

- **Take baby steps** Penetrative sex (i.e. intercourse) is often the most frightening part for both of you because: 1. Her "good girl" dilemmas rush to the fore; and 2. He requires an erection to do it. The more time you spend easing into it, doing everything but, the better. It gives his penis time to get past the shyness stage, plus if he's still phoning after pretty intense petting/oral sex sessions, she'll be reassured that he's not just in it for the sex.

- **Get the attitude right** Sex isn't a test. You're not going to be graded (and if it feels like you are, you're with the wrong person). So stop stressing and thinking "This has got to be just perfect." Sex is supposed to be fun! If it's feeling like you're about to take your road test, talk about it before going further. Say "I can't believe this, I've been waiting so long for this moment but I so want it to be right." If you're with the right person, they'll instantly jump in with reassurances. Perfect sex only happens on the soaps; normal people muddle through the first time.

GO!

- **Don't be a hero/heroine** If you're self-conscious, dim the lights or take your clothes off under the sheets.

- **Show how much you want them** Sincerity is sexy. Being genuinely turned on by someone is the biggest compliment of all. Let them know (even if their technique isn't perfect) that you're being sent to heaven simply because it's *their* hand/penis/tongue touching you.

- **Don't feel you have to perform like a trick pony** Working your way through an entire repertoire – ice cubes, chocolate sauce, positions an acrobat would have problems with – will only make it look like you're trying too hard. The slightly kinky/intense stuff can wait a little while. I'm not suggesting that you both stick to the missionary position (although it does tend to be the most favored position for first-time sex). But, aside from not knowing them well enough to define what's "kinky" and liable to freak them out, what's the rush?

- **Have a sense of humor** How you cope with a less-than-perfect performance can set the trend for your relationship. Even if the sex is disastrous, if you both laugh it off, snuggle up, and say "We'll do better next time," it really doesn't matter.

- **Resist the urge to say "How did I do?"** Remind yourself that really, really good sex invariably happens at least four to six sessions in. Try not to panic about it or the relationship (that's what next-day phone calls to friends are for). Hug, but not too tightly. There's a huge difference between lightly draping one of your limbs over theirs and clutching them like they're the last life raft on the *Titanic*.

What she's thinking

This is it then. Completely naked. Which is fine. Really. If I lie nice and flat, I'll keep a flat stomach and hide my butt at the same time. Except – ummm – this is feeling rather nice actually, so I'll just lie on my side so he can… Oh for God's sake, don't put your hand there! That's where all the fat's squashed up! Move it to…oooohh. That's more like it. Ummm. Where did he learn how to do that? So glad I'm not a guy though. It must be really smelly down there. Do I smell? Surely not. I had about 65 showers before he arrived. But I did have garlic last night. And Sandra said if you put a clove of garlic in your shoe, you'd smell it on your breath within two hours. Which means if you eat garlic, as opposed to stick a piece in your shoe, it's bound to…Oh God, he's good. Some girl's taught him this. Theres no way he'd figure it out on his own. Bet it's his ex Sarah. In fact, he's probably fantasizing about her right now. Bet she didn't eat garlic. Oooopphheeewwww. Phew! Ummm. Who cares, if he keeps on licking I'll marry him. Gosh. I think I'm about to.. I am…God, I don't usually…Oh hell, why is he stopping now? Oh, OK. No, no, it's fine. Ahem. This is it then. PleaseGod let those kegel exercises have worked. What if I'm not tight enough? What if he jokes about me to his friends. About there being enough room for a hot dog stand up there and everything. Must do more kegel… OH. MY. GOD! I'd forgotten how good this felt. Oh God. Oh God. Oh God. OH GOD…Oh… It's over. Too bad really…But look at his face! Poor thing. Better give him a hug. Or maybe he doesn't want one. He probably doesn't care what I think now. After all, he's had his way…and no way was I tight enough.

Bodytalk
Seduce with science

Here's a frightening thought: before you've even spoken to the person you've got your eye on, they've formed more than 80 percent of their first impression of you based solely on the way you walk and stand! We make what seem like outrageously snap judgments about people, but the fact is, almost every facet of our personality is shown in our appearance, posture, and the way we move. So how do you tell if your body is sending the right signals – and (more importantly) how do you read theirs? Let your body do the talking (and the flirting) by learning to recognize…

THE SEVEN SUREFIRE SIGNALS THAT SOMEONE IS FLIRTING WITH YOU

Eye contact We normally scan people's faces for three seconds – if they look for four and a half seconds, they're interested. To check: catch their gaze, hold it, then look away. Shy people often do a "Princess Di": they make eye contact, then, once they've caught you looking, drop their eyes and chin to the floor for a few seconds. Then they catch your eye again, by raising their eyes, chin tucked under. A wicked combination of vulnerability and blatant sexiness. And boy did she know it.

Smiling Start with small, quick smiles that light up your face like flashbulbs popping. Do this several times and catch their eye at the same time. Start smiling for longer periods. Then move into the "split-second delay" tactic: Don't smile immediately, instead look at their face for one long second. Look like you're really, really looking at them, then let a big, warm, beautiful smile take over your face. The split-second delay convinces people that your smile is genuine and meant only for them.

The flirting triangle When we look at people we're not close to, our eyes make a zigzag motion: we look from eye to eye and across the bridge of the nose. With friends, the look drops below eye level and moves into a triangle shape: we look from eye to eye but also look down to include the nose and mouth. Once we start flirting, the triangle gets even bigger – it widens at the bottom to include their good parts (like the body). Our eyes will start flickering downward to check out your chest (if you're a girl) and head farther south to where Dick lives (if you're a guy). Our gaze will then probably settle back on your mouth. If someone is watching your mouth while you're talking to them, it's very, very sexy because you can't help but wonder if they're imagining what it would be like to kiss you. Which is usually exactly what they are thinking, if they're looking intently at your mouth!

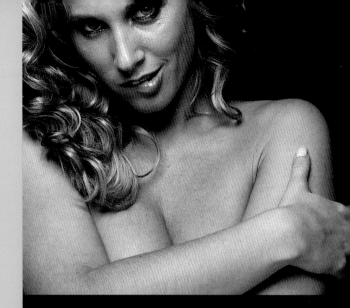

Mirroring This is what separates a good flirt from a great flirt: nothing will bond you more instantly or effectively. Mirroring simply means that you do whatever it is they do. If they lean forward, you lean forward. They sit back to take a sip of their drink, you do the same. We like people who are like us. If someone is doing what we're doing, we feel they're on the same level as us and in the same mood. Deliberately shift position and see if they follow.

The eyebrow flash When we first see someone we're attracted to, our eyebrows rise and fall. If they're attracted too, they'll raise their eyebrows in return. Never noticed? It's not surprising since the whole thing lasts about a fifth of a second! We're not consciously aware of doing it, but it's a gesture that is duplicated by every culture on earth. Watch for it if you meet someone new who you're attracted to. Tell them you're interested on a subconscious level by extending your eyebrow flash for up to a second – deliberately catching their eye for full impact. Sounds bizarre but you'll be convinced if you pay attention.

Pointing If we find someone attractive, we'll often point at them subconsciously with our hands, arms, legs, feet. Again, it's an unconscious way of making our intentions known. This is often picked up by the other person, unconsciously. So if you're got your eye on the hunk/babe in the corner, point your body in their direction – even if you don't make eye contact, they'll get the hint you're interested. In particular, point your feet their way.

Blinking If someone likes what they see, their pupil size increases and so does their blink rate. If you want to up the odds in your favor, try blinking more yourself. If the person likes you, they'll subconsciously try to match your blink rate to keep in sync. with you which, in turn, makes you both feel more attracted to each other!

The golden rule of body language

Don't ever judge on one thing alone. Sitting with your arms crossed often means that you're protecting yourself emotionally and shutting out the other person. Or it means you're freezing cold, having a fat day, or have just spilled coffee all over your top! Don't jump to conclusions; instead, look for clusters of behavior. If someone has their arms crossed and they're frowning and leaning backward to create as much space between the two of you as possible and their lips are pursed disapprovingly, it's a fairly safe bet you've done something to annoy the hell out of them. Most body language experts favor The Rule of Four, which means look for at least four body language signals that say the same thing before coming to a conclusion. Changes in body language also speak volumes – if she/he starts the evening by leaning in, resting their chin on their hands and gazing adoringly up at you and finishes it by leaning back, hands clasped in front of them like a severe schoolteacher, looking down their nose, you don't need me to tell you that the evening's not exactly been a roaring success. Keep an eye out for any dramatic changes in body language so you can fix any misunderstandings as they happen.

I've divided the following sections into tips for guys and tips for girls but quite frankly, both sections apply to both sexes, so you might want to read and learn from both. You never know what you might pick up!

SECRETS FOR BOYS: GET THE GIRL, GET YOUR HANDS ON HER BODY
Is it possible to read body language in a crowded, loud, busy bar? This is where reading body language truly comes into its own: it doesn't matter if it's a loud bar because you don't need to hear anything. All you need to do is watch. If it's crowded, get yourself into a position where you can see her as clearly as possible. Even if you can't see what's happening with the lower half of her body you can watch from the waist up. In really packed bars, stick to the obvious: eye contact and general signs. Is her body open to strangers (she's sitting relaxed with arms open)? Or has she closed herself off by crossing her arms tightly across her chest while sitting with a rigid spine? Is she smiling and looking friendly or frowning with an "Approach

Considering that it takes us between **ninety seconds** and **four minutes** to decide if we're attracted to someone, it's **pretty obvious** that attraction is not based on **witty one-liners**

me and I'll eat you (but not in the way you'd like)" expression? Is she making any preening gestures? The more she's fiddling with her clothes and hair, the more likely it is that she's trying to attract attention with her body.

OK, I think she's open to meeting someone and seems interested in me. What now? Do I need to walk over there? Keep your distance initially and instead make lots of eye contact. Wait until you're at the point where you're both constantly looking over, smiling, and catching each other's eyes. Rejection after this is highly unlikely (and after all, isn't that what this is all about? Not wanting to make a complete fool of yourself?). Then simply walk over and say "Hi. It's pretty obvious I can't stop looking at you so I thought I'd come and talk to you as well. Would you like a drink/dance/cigarette?" It's that simple! Forget the your-eyes-are-like-moonlight-reflected-off-the-wings-of-angels pick-up lines (but if you're going to use one, use that one). Considering that it takes us between ninety seconds and four minutes to decide if we're attracted to someone, it's pretty obvious that attraction is not based on witty one-liners. Fifty-five percent of the message we get from someone comes through body language. Thirty-eight percent is through the tone, speed, and inflection of the voice and a mere SEVEN percent through what is actually being said. So stop torturing yourself. Men sometimes think pick-up lines are crucial, when they're really not.

How do you tell when the woman you're dating is ready for sex? Classic giveaways: she'll hold eye contact while you're kissing. Move closer. Touch you a lot. Linger over the goodnight kiss and say "Ummmm" afterward while keeping her arms around your neck and fixing you with a wickedly flirtatious smile. If she's asked you over for dinner and there's candles, mood music, and she's wearing something that looks awfully easy to slip off, it's a pretty safe bet she's hoping you'll get intimate (assuming her mother's not in the next room). Another "girl" trick that tells you it's safe to pass go: she'll sit back on the sofa and put her legs in your lap. If you start stroking her calves, then move farther up her leg to her thighs and she doesn't flinch, it's looking good. If you

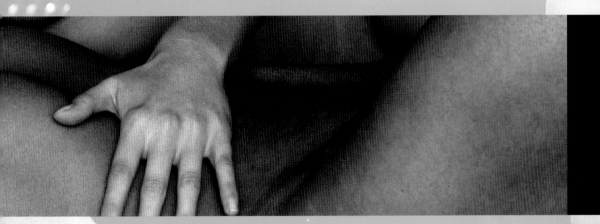

start kissing her at this point and she responds passionately, it's OK to start caressing her shoulders, then move on to her breasts. If you've had your hands underneath her top and bra and she doesn't put her clothes back in order when you both come up for air, it's the equivalent of her saying, "Keep going." Having said all that, I still strongly recommend that you check you've interpreted her body language correctly by backing it up with words.

Is it better to come out and tell her you want her or do you just trust body language? Body language speaks volumes, but to ensure that you've read the signs correctly, simply say, "Oh God. Can I keep going?" or "Do you want to move into the bedroom?" Don't be surprised if she says "Not sure" but then dives in for another tongue-down-the-tonsils kiss which makes you think she'd like your tongue inserted elsewhere. It's the nice-girls-don't thing at work and she's looking for reassurance that you don't think she's a hussy for wanting sex as much as you do. (Yes, girls are confusing.) Switch to "God, you're beautiful/gorgeous/soooooo sexy" and say things like, "OK. But I just love touching you so much." and she'll get the message you don't think she's a "bad girl" for wanting it as much as you do. (HUGE warning here. If she says "I'm not sure" and sits back, take her at her word. She means it – do not proceed at any cost. Needless to say if she says "No," it means No. Keep going and you'll be up for rape – with me testifying for her.)

SECRETS FOR GIRLS: 11 FABULOUS CLUES TO HELP YOU FIND MR. RIGHT (FOR NOW)

So much of what he does speaks volumes about the kind of guy he is or is likely to be. All of these gestures and signals give away much more than you'd think. So keep your eyes open and learn to read between the lines…

He's a face-fiddler People tend to touch their noses or cover their mouths when they're lying. When we were little children, we'd clap both hands over our mouths whenever we told a lie. It's an immature attempt to put the words "back in." As adults, we realize that this gesture gives the game away, so we stop doing it. Or we try to anyway. Subconsciously, the gesture has been learned so our hands still shoot toward our faces when we lie. All we can do then is to disguise it by pretending we're scratching our noses or touching our faces. So you want to figure out if they really are single? If they look away, their hand touches their nose, and they look down to the floor while fidgeting, it's a pretty safe bet that they're telling lies. People also use distracting body language to divert your attention. They'll choose that moment to fiddle with the cuffs on their shirt, or look at their wrists and palms. If their palms are facing upward and their wrists are exposed they're not hiding anything. People find it extremely difficult to lie with their palms open and upward.

He's a dog owner He's used to putting other's needs first (like yours) and used to dealing with doggy drools and shedding hair, so he's unlikely to be a hygiene freak (the ultimate turn-off in bed). Also pay attention to the breed of dog he's chosen. It's a foaming-at-the-mouth-straining-at-the-leash Rottweiller/Alsation/Fang-bearing Scary Thing? Love me, love my dog means he admires the qualities his canine possesses, i.e. this guy's into exhibitionistic shows of masculinity (otherwise known as the small man or small penis syndrome). Even the kindest interpretation means he's a man in a hurry – not really a great bet for slow, sensual foreplay. If it's a preened poodle at the end of the leash, he could be the other extreme and a little *too* in touch with his feminine side. Best bet of all: the man tugging along the cute mutt. Not only does this show a healthy lack of regard for looks and a huge respect for charisma (yes, dogs have it too!), but it also means he's capable of looking beyond the obvious to find any not-so-obvious sexy qualities.

He's not Brad Pitt If he's not amazingly great-looking, he's not inundated with women pressing their bodies against his. So it's likely he'll spend time and effort keeping the ones that do happy.

He smells…divine Smell is one of the indicators of attraction and the better he smells to you, the more genetically complementary the two of you may be.

He's erect Get your mind out of the gutter! I mean standing up straight! Bad posture is indicative of laziness. If he stands with his shoulders back and his tummy in, it means he's not a slouch and will probably make an effort in bed. Good posture also screams confidence.

He's funny Anyone who can laugh at himself out of bed, is going to be unselfconscious in it. Self-deprecating humor is a great sign that he doesn't take himself too seriously and isn't egocentric.

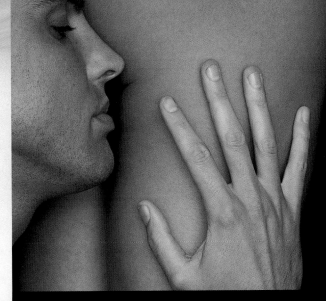

He's bilingual It's a complete myth that the French/Italians are better lovers than the rest of us, but it's a very good sign if he speaks more than one language. It's a sign of intelligence and effort: he's willing to work hard for rewards. A great sign in a long-term lover!

How's his driving? He's impatient and suffers from road rage? Forget it! He'll be an impatient lover who's obsessed with the final destination (orgasm – his) and uninterested in the journey (usually when you get yours). If he's a fast driver, fasten your seat belt but go along for the ride: it usually means he's passionate and into lusty, wanton sex. Steer clear of cautious, slower-than-your-granny type drivers – even she'd want more action!

How's his walk? If he walks superfast, he's got places to go, people to meet, and a sense of purpose. This will translate one of two ways in bed: he'll either be incredibly impatient, switch positions 65 billion times per session, and think all roads lead to intercourse. Or he'll be confident and adventurous: which translates into a willingness to experiment. Whichever, he's likely to be the type to have sex all over the house rather than just in the bedroom.

What's his routine? If he's so set in his routine, he hyperventilates when forced to catch the 6:05 instead of the 6:03 train, then it's worrying sexually. He's robotic and reeks of predictability: chances are he makes love in exactly the same way every single time (and don't even think about moving an inch to the left or he'll wonder what's wrong). And while it's fine to stick to what you're good at, it does help if he's flexible enough to accommodate to your needs.

Attached at the hip – to his friends. If he only moves as one of the crowd, he'll be a nervous lover. He'd need lots of encouragement before he'd relax as he's probably not terribly good at thinking for himself. If you know what you want, he'll fit in with you. But don't expect any surprises: he's too scared to take a risk and veer into unchartered kingdoms.

Hand signals

- **Talking with his hands** If he's using big, sweeping, dramatic movements, it probably translates well into the bedroom. It usually means that he's imaginative and creative and will want sex to be a "production". See if he measures up to the ultimate sex flex by pulling his thumb: the more flexible the hand, the more adventurous he is. If you can hardly pull his thumb away from the main body of the palm, he's a straight, conservative lover. The further it flexes, the more bent he becomes. Take a good look at it while you're there: a large or long and heavy thumb means he's got vast amounts of sexual energy and likes to take control. Short thumbs aren't great (weak-willed) but thumbs set very low on his hand are – this guy's sexually unconventional and highly adventurous. Yummy!

- **Nail-noshing** Nail-biters push themselves to the limits (hence the stress-busting biting habit) by pushing boundaries and going to extremes. Which usually equates to passion.

- **Loopy handwriting** According to handwriting experts, people who sign a lower-case "y" with a flourish in the tail allegedly have high libidos and lots of imagination.

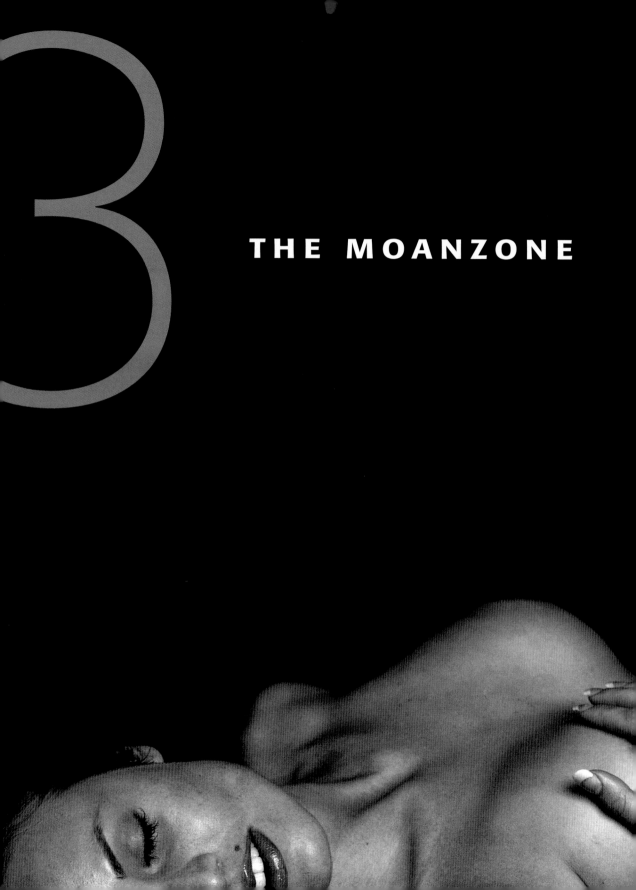

3

THE MOANZONE

The **really dirty stuff**: hands-on hints on mutual masturbation, the all-time ultimate guide to giving **great oral** sex, plus **tricks and trivia** to turn you both into penis geniuses!

Oh. My. God.
The definitive guide to oral sex

When researchers asked a group of college kids which they'd pick if forced to give up either intercourse or oral sex, both sexes gave penetration the heave-ho. I'm with them. As much as a hard, throbbing erection is desperately appealing, a soft, warm tongue is damn near irresistible. Let's face it: find the person whose mouth makes all the right moves and join the line of those eager to lap up the attention. The opposite also applies: refuse to get up close and personal and don't be surprised if your dancecard stays permanently empty.

Why? Not only is oral sex one of life's great pleasures, but our attitude toward it speaks volumes about our attitude to sex in general. Open, uninhibited, sensuous lovers adore both giving and receiving oral. Prissy, uptight, and why-would-you-possibly-want-to-go-there are adjectives which apply to the rest of the population. Eager to learn a few more tricks to add to your existing repertoire? I suspect you'll find a couple here. Your grandmother probably told you the way to a lover's heart is through his stomach. Well, try heading south a bit. There's guides for both of you, but ladies first…

THE LICK OF LOVE: MAGICAL MOUTH TECHNIQUES FOR HER
Trim and terrific Encourage her to trim any excess pubic hair or have it waxed. The less hair around the clitoris, the greater the pleasure for both of you (coughing up an errant hair like a cat with a fur ball isn't sexy). While she's doing her part, do yours by shaving just before you nuzzle around down there. Stubble leaves a rash and it *hurts*.

Don't take a nosedive Ripping back the covers and diving straight for it isn't a turn-on. Anticipation is everything. Work your way down her body – kissing, nibbling, licking nipples, tummy, thighs – and make her wait. Her hips should be straining upward in a (vain) attempt to hurry things up before you take it any further. Like, you're oh-so-close it's ridiculous. And while we're on the subject of being up close and personal, a healthy vagina shouldn't smell unpleasant. If hers does, she may have an infection or need to make some diet adjustments. Which is why a garlic-laden dinner *à deux* in that romantic French restaurant isn't such a great idea if you want to do more than just hold hands afterward. Yup, it doesn't just show up on her breath.

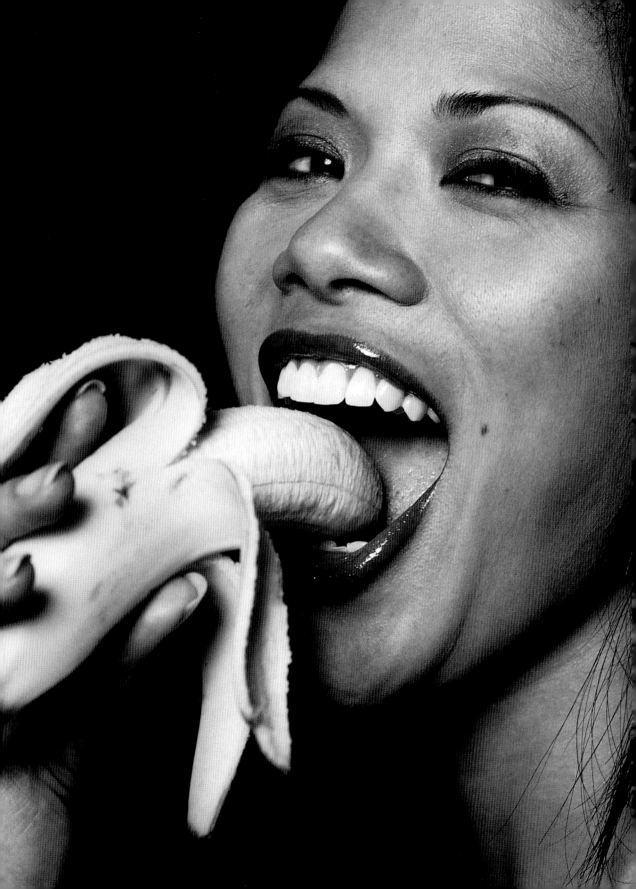

Get a head start Let her demonstrate what tongue technique she'd like you to use by getting her to lick your palm the way she'd like you to lick her. She'll probably use the whole flat of her tongue rather than a tensed tip, and wiggle and swish in a slow, lazy, large movement.

Power positions
- Her on top: instead of her lying back and you lying between her legs, you lie back on the bed and get her to climb on top of you, facing the headboard. She puts her hands against the wall behind the bed to steady herself, then lowers onto your mouth and tongue. This gives her complete control over the pressure: she can lift away from your mouth if it's too rough, move close if she wants it harder. Your neck's not cramped and it stops your tongue from getting as tired. (A comfort tip for other positions: If she's on her side you can rest your head on her thigh.)
- Through the roof: she lies back on the bed, you kneel between her legs, then you lift them up so they're resting on your shoulders. You're in a kneeling position, she's lifted in the air, her shoulders still on the bed. She uses her hands to support herself, plus you're supporting her by holding her legs. This feels fantastic and she gets the added turn-on of seeing exactly what's going on.

Keep it covered Get her to leave her underwear on and start by licking through the fabric. (Yes, it helps if she's wearing satin or silk, rather than the graying thick cotton numbers.) Instead of removing them completely to finish the job, pull them to one side. This will transport her straight back to her first oral experiences (when she was young, trying hard to be good – and failing spectacularly).

Making mouth music Separate the vaginal lips with your fingers, find her clitoris (a tiny marble at the top end – the end near her stomach – covered with a hood of skin), and make gentle, upward strokes around the clitoris, not on it. Use the flat of your tongue, not the tip. Keep your tongue relaxed and not only will she like it better, but also you'll be able to lick her longer. Make slow circles around the circumference and combine this with an up-and-down, lapping motion. Let as much of your tongue as possible make contact so you're covering the largest area possible. Practice on your own palm and see which movements feel most efficient. If you notice her clitoris shrinking or retracting back under the hood of skin, you're being too rough.

Direct directions When you're in position, it's difficult to interpret anything but moaning and the most simple sentences. After all, her legs are covering your ears and emerging to ask "What did you say?" isn't ideal when it was "For God's sake, don't stop because I'm just about to…". Ask her to use single-word instructions like "lighter," "harder," "perfect." She may also use body language to show you what she wants. If she pulls your head closer or rises up to meet you, she wants you to go harder. If she's wriggling away, you're being too rough or too fast.

V marks the spot If you're having trouble hitting the hot spot, ask her to guide you to the right place by forming a "V" with her fingers, positioning them where she wants you to focus. You lick between them.

Take sides According to some sexperts, one side of the clitoris is often more pleasure-prone than the other. See if this holds true for her: make her clitoris more accessible by getting her to keep her left leg bent at the knee and angled outward while straightening the right one so it's in line with her body. Then switch legs.

Write a love letter Use your tongue like a pen and "write" on her clitoris, spelling out each letter of whatever sentences you've made up in your head. This ensures you're varying your movements and means you won't overstimulate one particular area.

Bring up the rear Spread your hands wide and grip her bottom firmly. Squeeze and start rotating in big, wide circles. This feels good because it indirectly stimulates the anal area – a highly sensitive area for women as well as men, although some women are a little shy about admitting this. This does the job, without her feeling uncomfortable. (Plenty of women aren't shy and like a finger inserted into their anus as well as vagina on orgasm, but ask first and use lots of lubricant.)

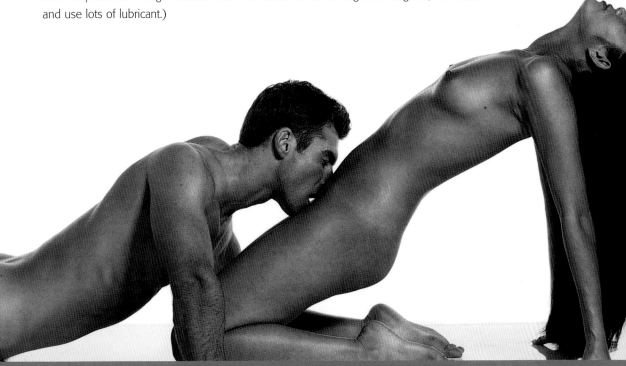

Lots of women stay absolutely still during orgasm. **Others gyrate** like they're **lap dancing for Latvia.** Keep going regardless. Many men stop licking at **the crucial moment,** thinking it's all over.

Don't be a show-off   Switching techniques might score you points in the early stages, but stick to one technique once she approaches orgasm.

Lift off   Increase the speed and pressure but keep on doing whatever it is you're doing and keep the rhythm regular. Lots of women stay absolutely still during orgasm. Others gyrate like they're lap dancing for Latvia. Keep going regardless. Our orgasms last ages and many men stop licking at the crucial moment, thinking it's all over. Well, it may be for you if you get it wrong! Keep on with slow, gentle strokes until she pushes you away. (Which she may well do because the clitoris gets extremely sensitive after orgasm, so don't be offended!)

BLOW HIS...MIND: TIPS AND TRICKS TO TAKE HIM TO HEAVEN
The visual feast   Leave the lights on so he can see what you're doing. Give him real front-row action by tying your hair back as well. If you're brave, hold eye contact while you're fellating him; if you're too embarrassed, look at his penis instead.

Position-plus
- He stands, you sit facing him on the side of the bed (or on a piece of furniture that's the right height). It's more comfortable for both of you and it leaves your hands free to stimulate his penis, nipples, testicles, perineum, etc., and they won't get cramped. It also gives you control over how deeply he thrusts into your mouth. Some men say their legs go weak on orgasm but most can survive if they collapse on the bed immediately afterward!
- He stands, you kneel in front of him. It's more comfortable than lying down beside him though the chief appeal is your classic "submissive" pose. (If being on your knees reeks so much of subservience your feminist friends would never forgive you, ditch the friends, not the position!)

But not yet...   Lick your way downward until his penis is straining for attention, then bypass it completely by licking down the outside of his thighs until you reach the inside of his knee, then move back up his inner thigh until you get to his testicles. Stop right there and drive him nuts, using large tongue movements to swirl around each testicle.

Add hands   Get the hand motion under control before you add your mouth. If he's not circumsized, don't tug or yank at the foreskin, manipulate it so it slides up and over the head and, again, remember to keep things nice and slippery. Use your hands, not your mouth, to control his penis and always use two hands. One holds the penis so it doesn't move all over, the other touches him elsewhere. It also takes the pressure off – literally – if you alternate between two kinds of stimulation simultaneously.

Liquid licks   Before you head downward, let lots of saliva pool in your mouth (sorry, far too much information I know, but I did promise to tell you everything!). It really can't be too wet for him inside there, so keep some water close by if your mouth gets dry. The more lubricated he is, the more pleasurable it will feel.

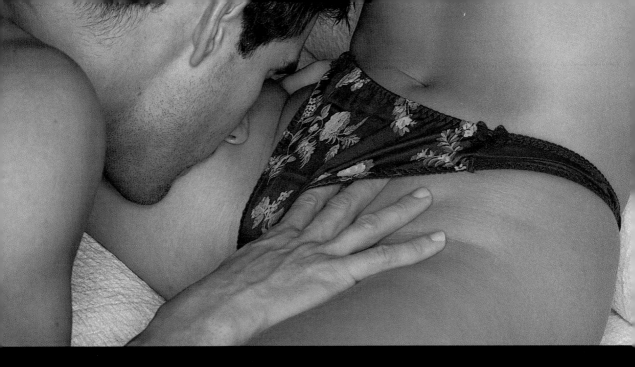

Ripping back the covers and diving straight for it, isn't a turn-on. **Anticipation is everything.** Work your way down her body – kissing, nibbling, licking nipples, stomach, thighs – and **make her wait.**

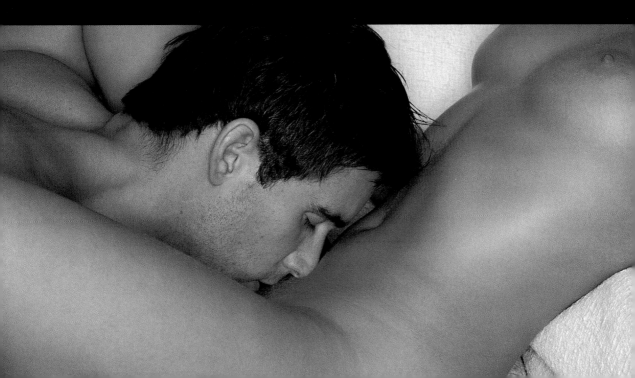

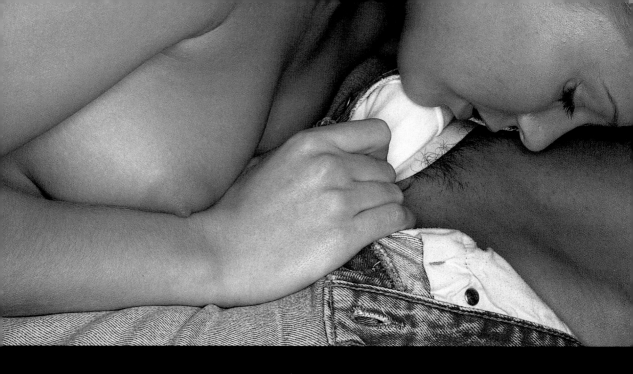

Contrary to popular belief, **semen is not sulfuric acid**, but you'd think it was considering the way some women go on about it! It **tastes** a little **like alfafa sprouts**.

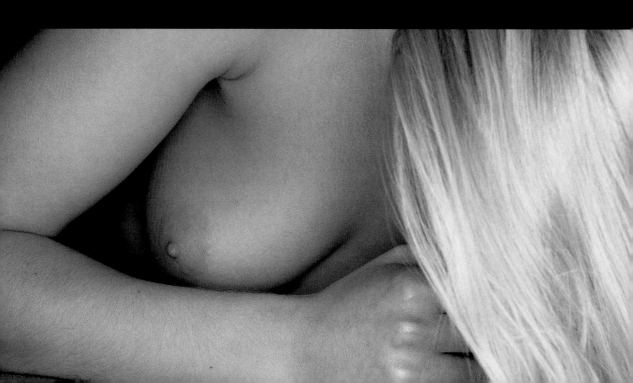

Oral action Go lower for a lollipop lick – one fabulously long lick from the base of his penis right to the top – then make an "O," and in one movement, slide your mouth over his erection, taking him as far in as is comfortable. Move from there into the bread-and-butter stroke: with one hand, grip the bottom of the shaft while you slide your mouth up and down. The basic hand movement stays the same: slide your hand up and down, closing it when you reach the head, opening it slightly as you slide down the length. Establish a regular fellatio rhythm, then move into the twist-and-swirl. Make a twisting motion with one hand as you're sliding up and down and swirl your tongue around the rim of the head, paying particular attention to the frenulum (the skin on the underside of his penis tip).

Access all areas Keep stimulating other areas while you're fellating him. Try firmly stroking (or massaging in minicircles) the perineum (the area between his anus and testicles). Tickle and stroke the area below his belly button and the base of his penis just as he's about to orgasm.

On the home run As with women, it's important that you maintain a steady rhythm to build excitement. As he approaches orgasm, however, step up the speed and pressure.

The fellatio finale If you don't want to finish him off in your mouth, switch to intercourse just before the crucial moment. The next best thing to you swallowing: using your hands to masturbate him and letting him orgasm over your breasts.

My pleasure Now all that's left to do is…lie back and wait for the congratulations. They should follow immediately after he's finished moaning "Oh. My. God." about 25 times.

I hate giving oral! Do I really have to do it?

The short answer is yes. Refuse to give a guy oral and he has every right to get it elsewhere (and the same applies to you). It's one of the most pleasurable aspects of sex and to deny him it and expect him to remain faithful is unthinkable. Besides, there are three main reasons why women don't like giving men oral sex. Happily each has a very simple solution…

- **It smells** Have a shower together beforehand or ask him to. If he's not circumsized, make sure he pulls back the foreskin and washes beneath.

- **I gag** Change your position and technique for maximum control. Get him to stand in front of you, while you sit on the bed facing him. Use one hand to control his penis, placing it at the bottom of the shaft, and you're now in the ultimate position to control how deeply you take him into your mouth. Most feeling is in the head of the penis, not the shaft, so you don't need to go too deep. If he does that charming hands-behind-your-head-to-shove-you-down-further thing, tell him if he does it again, you'll not just stop immediately but permanently.

- **Swallowing makes me want to throw up** If you don't want to swallow, don't! Instead, continue stimulating him with your hand and let him ejaculate elsewhere on your body. Contrary to popular belief, semen is not sulfuric acid, but you'd think it was considering the way some women go on about it! It tastes a little like alfalfa sprouts that still have some dirt clinging to them. Not quite chocolate but hardly disgusting. (And if his is, he needs to look at his diet and cut out the beer, chips, spicy foods, and garlic.) Another trick if you don't like the taste: swallow it quickly and in one gulp, the way you do medicine.

Hands on!

A supersexy guide to
giving great "hand"

As overexcited teenagers, a French kiss and someone's hand fiddling around "down there" was enough to make us faint with pleasure. Then along came oral sex and intercourse and both kissing and hand stimulation got crossed off the agenda in favor of supposedly superior sensations. Big mistake. Not only is it silly to narrow our sexual repertoire rather than expand it, but the humble old hand-job also has several distinct advantages over the competition.

Feeling fat and unattractive? You don't need to remove your clothes and get naked to give him what he's asking for. Got your period? If you're squeamish but horny, leave the tampon in and let him give you an orgasm by using his fingers on your clitoris. Engrossed in a movie and want to do it and her simultaneously? Keep those eyes glued to the screen and let your fingers do the walking. You don't need condoms because it's almost totally safe sex (unless you've got cuts on your hands/penis/vagina, the risk of passing on infection is extremely low). It's a great way of dabbling sexually with a new partner until you're ready for the intimacy of oral sex or penetration.

And you're much more likely to get away with doing it in public: he's driving and stuck in traffic/you're on a plane with her, a blanket over both your laps. Hand sex also paves the way for other diversionary delights. If his penis is starting to feel left out, invite him in to play. The head is wonderfully soft and ideal for stimulating the ultrasensitive clitoris. (It's softer than a baby's bottom – I swear it!) Use your hands to guide it up and down, stroking over the entire clitoral area for a high-voltage velvety vibe!

A hand down our pants evokes innocent but steamy memories of Bobby or Betty behind the bleachers at school and, last but not least, a hand-job feels heavenly. With one hand on your genitals, another caressing elsewhere, a tongue in your mouth, and lips pressed against yours, you're drowning in a sea of sensations because you're getting it from all sides, all at once. Ready to revamp an old classic into your new favorite thing? Keep reading…

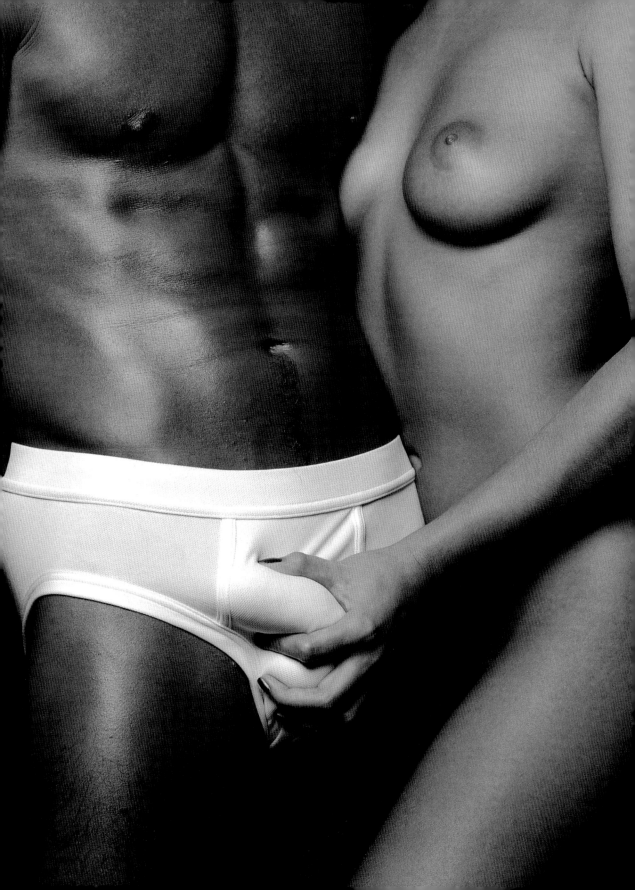

HIS TURN

Alex Comfort (aka Mr. *Joy of Sex*) says a woman who knows how to masturbate a man "subtly, unhurriedly, and mercilessly" will almost always make a superlative partner. I thoroughly agree – and suspect Mr. Comfort would approve of this step-by-step guide.

- **Err, how do I do this again?** Don't be embarrassed to admit that you don't have a clue what you're doing – he'll be more than happy to demonstrate. Unlike some holier-than-thou women who claim they can't show their boyfriends how they like to be touched because they've never masturbated (wide eyes, batting lashes – oh puhleeze!), you'd be hard-pressed to find a man who won't admit he's been doing it since age seven. Get him to show you what rhythm, speed, and pressure he likes by putting your hand over his as he masturbates himself. When you think you've got it figured out, swap hands so your hand's now underneath and his is on top. Ask for feedback if you're doing it right. If he's too shy, hand-feed him by asking: "harder?/faster?/slower?" and look for a nod or shake of the head.

This won't just **take him to heaven;** he'll be driven there by a **big-busted blonde** in a **Ferrari.**

- **Use lubricant** Sometimes a combination of saliva and pre-ejaculatory fluid (the stuff that comes out before orgasm when he's excited) is enough to keep things nice and slippery. It's always a good idea, though, to keep a tube of personal lubricant near the bed. A dry hand-job is OK. A wet one won't just take him to heaven; he'll be driven there by a big-busted blonde in a Ferrari.
- **Get comfy** Forget lying beside him on the bed. Instead, straddle his chest and face toward his penis, or get him to kneel on the bed in front of you, or stand in front of the bed while you sit on it. All three positions mean you can use both hands without losing balance and touch other areas. Plus you'll be more inclined to take time and really spoil him if you're in a comfortable position.
- **The basic stroke** Use one hand to hold the penis steady, and the other to slide up and down the shaft in a whole-hand, loose-fist movement, closing your fist gently but firmly as it slides up and over the head. The technique is roughly the same whether he's circumcised or not, but you've got more to work with if it's intact. Never, EVER, yank the foreskin back until he's properly lubricated (unless you *want* to cause him pain!). Use saliva or lubricant to make it nice and slippery, then gently ease the foreskin back and over the head of the penis, "rolling" it down the shaft. You can then work with the foreskin, sliding it up and over the head during the basic stroke.
- **Get the pressure right** Too gentle can feel like "nothing," but too firm HURTS!!!! If in doubt, start off gently and ask him if it's hard enough. It's easy to get a little carried away once you get into the swing of it. If you're starting to think of his penis as a big bendy plaything and at the point where

you're wondering if you could twist it to make an animal, like they do with balloons, stop right there! Penises are human flesh and – even more surprising – attached to an owner! (Yes, he is still there!)

- **Feel the rhythm** Start off s-l-o-w and t-e-a-s-i-n-g-l-y tortuous, then speed up as he moves toward orgasm. Going too fast too soon usually does one of two things (neither is great): 1. He becomes insensitive to your touch; 2. He gets sore and becomes oversensitive. A good hand-job is like a good movie. It starts off slowly and interesting, then builds steadily to a glorious climax – with interesting twists and turns along the way.

- **My hand's about to fall off!** Removing both hands and massaging them while saying "Owww!" and rocking back and forth isn't the sexiest sight in the world. Besides, you can't just leave him, well, hanging. Instead, give your fingers a rest by simply wrapping them around his penis, holding firm and holding still. Give each hand a rest in this way. Even if you're not feeling numb or tired, stopping for a minute or so can up the tension nicely, so don't feel guilty!

- **What now? Looks like he's about to…!** It's all individual, but most men prefer that you increase pressure and rhythm significantly the few seconds before orgasm, then slow it down and be gentler during it. Just don't stop completely! After orgasm, a lot of men are ultrasensitive: that loving squeeze could have him shooting through the roof rather than leaning over for a smooch. Most important, though, don't fuss over the cleanup. If I EVER catch ANY of you doing that girly, eeww-how-messy-is-this thing, your supersexpert status will be withdrawn immediately!

A twist on the usual

- **Be a boy scout** Place his penis in between your two flat palms, fingers extended so that your hands are straight. Now roll them as if his penis were pastry. It's great if he's got erection problems, and yummy even if not.

- **Run rings around him** Make sure he's well-lubricated, then make two rings around his penis with the thumb and index finger of each hand. Place them next to each other in the middle of the shaft, then continually slide in opposite directions simultaneously.

- **Play Twister** Triple the sensation of the basic stroke by twisting your hand as you reach the part where the head meets the shaft. This applies extra stimulation to the frenulum (the area of puckered skin on the underside of the penis), which is packed with nerve endings and supersensitive.

- **The minimassage** Here, you're using the same technique you would to massage his back but on a much smaller area. Start with both thumbs placed in the middle of the base of his penis on the underside (the side closest to his testicles). Now gently push your thumbs, massaging upward and outward, always returning to the center and working up the shaft as you go.

- **Tease please** Build up to a constant rhythm, then every few minutes slow it down and ease the pressure to frustratingly light for 10 seconds. Repeat at least four times.

- **Pull his hair** Tug gently but rhythmically on his pubic hair, starting by gently pulling a few strands between your thumb and forefinger, then pulling larger amounts. Because his penis extends inside, as well as out, this massages the internal part.

HER TURN

Men are usually better at giving hand-jobs to women because they've had more practice: all that time at "second base," trying desperately to turn your girlfriend on so she'll finally give in and go "all the way" has paid off. If you're still a little uncertain, take a tip from Britain's bad boy, *FHM* magazine's sexpert Grub Smith. He instructs his male readers to "do everything half as fast and twice as softly as you think you should." Keep this as your hands-on mantra, combine it with the following, and you can't go wrong.

- **Leave her hat on** Double the delight by leaving her clothes on for as long as possible. Fondle and stroke her breasts through a sheer slippery bra before moving on to stroke her clitoris through sexy underwear. Not only does it give her even more incentive to invest in grrrrreat lingerie (seems worth it if it's not ripped off immediately), it's a huge turn-on when you finally do push aside the material to touch naked flesh.

- **The warm up** Before you even think about paddling toward the little man in the boat (the clitoris, in case you're wondering), try cupping the whole vulva (genital area) through her clothes and gently applying even, circular pressure. Keep the fabric of her undies between you, then try placing your first and middle fingers in between her labia lips lengthways and vibrating them in a gentle scissor motion.

- **Get into position** The usual technique involves reaching one hand down while kissing or lying beside her. A far more practical – albeit not as romantic – position is to sit facing her between her open legs, while she's either sitting or lying back with her knees up. Try her positioned on a chair/the side of the bed/kitchen counter, with you kneeling or sitting in front.

- **Stroke her thighs** One at a time – fingers splayed and trailing up her inner thighs then over her vagina but not lingering – then use both hands to stroke up both thighs simultaneously. Keep going until her legs open wider and wider and it's obvious she wants you to center on her genital region.

- **Let her do the work** Start by holding your fingers against her closed labia and pay attention to how she positions herself and grinds against you. This is your clue to where she wants you to concentrate and how much pressure she requires. At all times her hip movements – how fast and how furiously she grinds them against your hand – are your guide to the pressure and speed she's craving. If she's not grinding against your hand at all, you're either doing it perfectly (gold star!) or she's unsure of how you'll react if she gives you feedback. All the more reason to…

- **Ask for help** While reading her hip movements helps, if you think she's up for it, much better to ask her to show you how she masturbates. The usual lesson you'll learn from this if she obliges: it's better to run your finger around the clitoris than stimulate it directly. While we're on the topic, just as you hate her going straight for the family jewels, it's also a really, really bad idea to ignore the labia lips and rush straight for the main attraction: the clitoris. If the clitoris is stimulated too early, too hard, or too soon, the reaction you'll get is more likely to be pain than pleasure.

- **Getting technical** OK, now we're ready to (ahem) dive straight in. But first, test how lubricated she is by gently running one finger along the crease of the labia lips. Don't be put off if she's not sliding off the bed already. It could mean you're not turning her on or need to prolong foreplay, but everything from the taking the Pill to a yeast infection can also affect how wet she is. Quite often, the lubrication is there, it's just trapped inside. If you gently insert a fingertip inside the vagina, you can spread the lubrication around (but not directly on) the clitoris.

- **Go for it** This is a variation on the "cupping" we did earlier. Place your palm over her pubic hair and bend your middle finger so it's angled to touch her clitoris. Cup her pubic area and use your finger to rub her clitoris up and down or in circles. Slide the two fingers next to it alongside so they stimulate the edges of the labia. Next, use your middle finger to make circles or figure eights around the clitoris. Your main stroke now involves touching and rubbing the shaft of the clitoris – the part behind the clitoral hood (the skin which protects and covers the clitoris). Although most action does center around the clitoris, it's a rare woman who can cope with direct and prolonged stimulation on it.

- **The two golden rules** Rule No 1: DON'T change technique, especially when she's heading straight for the "Oooooowwwwweeeeeeeee" stage. You think showing off an infinite variety of hand twirls will result in her saying, "Wow! You know so many ways to use your fingers! What a star!" It won't. She'll fix you with a look of rage and/or frustration (probably both) and say "What were you trying to prove? If you'd just kept on doing it the one way, it would have worked. Why did you have to be such a show-off?" Well, even if she smiles sweetly and pretends to be happy, believe me – that's what she wanted to say. So think one method, one speed. The only thing that should interrupt the flow is if she's not flowing: the one thing she won't mind you stopping for is to lubricate the area. In case you hadn't guessed, that's Rule No 2: Keep things wet. It's impossible for her to be too wet, but oh-so-easy to be too dry. The minute you feel lubrication starting to dry up, add more. Another dollop of lubricant or lots of saliva.

- **But what happened to bringing her to orgasm simply by thrusting inside with my fingers?** Women don't usually masturbate by thrusting a finger in and out of their vaginas, so there's not much point in you trying to make them orgasm by using just the same technique, is there boys? Combine it with clitoral stimulation if you want to tip her over the edge.

What happens to your body during sex?

A four-step guide to the sexual response cycle

While you're moaning, groaning, and lying back enjoying the ride, your body's checking off a massive to-do list to make it all happen. The brain hones in on the pleasurable sensations, while your sexual system works its butt off to create all the physiological changes necessary for arousal or orgasm.

The sexual response cycle roughly divides into four phases – and you can thank sex pioneers Masters and Johnson for researching them. As always, knowledge is power. Understand the theory of what's happening inside the pleasure zone and you're one step ahead of the rest. PS: Don't get too hung up if your body doesn't do what it's "supposed to," or deviates from the order.

THE EXCITEMENT PHASE

Nipples harden and become erect, breathing quickens, the skin may become flushed.
Him: Blood flows into the penis, making it swell; the testicles begin to flatten and rise. As excitement increases, a drop of pre-ejaculatory fluid comes out of the top of the penis, nicely lubricating the area.
Her: The vaginal walls contract, causing a secretion of fluid that lubricates the vagina. Blood flows to the clitoris, making it enlarge, harden, and protrude from between the vaginal lips.

THE PLATEAU PHASE

Heart rate, breathing, blood pressure, muscular tension – all start to skyrocket.
Him: The penis reaches its maximum size, the testicles flatten and rise even closer to the body. This is the point where men need to stop stimulation immediately or be totally unable to control ejaculation.
Her: The vagina expands while contractions and lubrication increase. Increased blood flow to the labia and vaginal entrance cause the whole area to darken to a deep red/purple color.

THE ORGASMIC PHASE

The nipples are erect, a slight reddening appears across the chest and genitals, the heart speeds up, the body's muscles tense, and the anus also contracts. While the feeling of orgasm is spectacular, the process of it is relatively simple. Sex therapist Carole Altman's explanation is the best I've read: orgasm happens when the genital area cannot stand the increased blood flow. The body then "lets go" and the blood flows back to the rest of the body. It's this instant release – the spasm of letting the blood rush back to the rest of the body and the release of muscular tension – that is the orgasm.

Him: The seminal vesicle is full and semen begins to flow upward, toward the head of the penis. This moment is called "ejaculatory inevitability." You could wave a million dollars in front of him and he'd still be powerless to stop. The penis contracts once every 0.8 of a second and semen spurts out of the tip. Orgasm and ejaculation are two separate processes: ejaculation is the physical part; orgasm the feeling.

Her: The entire genital area is engorged with blood and the clitoris is erect. On climax, lubrication increases dramatically and the vaginal walls contract once every 0.8 of a second – the same interval as his penile contractions. (To help make up for his orgasms being more automatic and easier to attain, however, Mother Nature kindly extends the length of female sensation. His orgasm usually lasts an average of five seconds; hers lasts about 15.) The uterus contracts and dips down slightly during orgasm. This also causes the mouth of the cervix to dip – directly into the vaginal cavity where he's spilled his semen, giving it a head start on the long journey to the egg.

THE RESOLUTION PHASE

The body returns to "normal." Blood drains from the genitals; heart rate and blood pressure decrease.

Him: The testicles drop and become looser and larger. The penis returns to half its erect size immediately and to its normal size within 30 minutes. Few men can go straight from resolution to the excitement or orgasm phase immediately. Most men need a resting stage after orgasm, when the body relaxes and rejuvenates itself, refusing to become aroused until it's achieved both.

Her: The blood flows away from the genital area and the genitals lose their heightened color. The clitoris often feels extremely sensitive immediately after orgasm. Why? One minute it's engorged with blood, the next it's drained of it – so it's gone from one extreme to the other. This is also the reason why skin can often feel itchy post-orgasm.

How to spot if someone's just gotten some

Think your dinner party hostess got more than dessert when she disappeared into the kitchen just now? Learn to spot the telltale signs of recent sexual activity and you'll soon see if it's more than the oven that made her hot. In fact…

It's blinking obvious Check out her eyes to see if she's blinking rapidly: both our blinking and breathing rate speed up right after sex. The day after sex, however, we'll blink less frequently and more slowly than someone who wasn't quite so lucky the night before.

She's got the glow A brisk walk in the fresh air will bring a healthy glow to the cheeks – but so will a good old romp in the sack. Around 30 percent of women experience visible post-coital glow. Because arousal causes an increase in blood pressure that lasts around 20 minutes after orgasm, our lips also swell and look bigger and redder (all the more reason to swap the surgeon, with a big, scary collagen injection, for a boyfriend, with a big, sexy erection).

Her toes tell a story Bizarre but true: the little toe on the left foot turns red after you've just had sex – or even if you're just thinking about it. The spacing of our toes give other clues. Our little toe represents sex, the one next to it love. Got a gap between the two? You're a fan of casual sex. A little toe that twists toward the fourth means you might be gay or bisexual.

She looks fantastic People who enjoy regular, frequent sex tend to sport lustrous-looking hair, clear, shiny eyes, great muscle tone, and general good health. They're also the last to catch colds, the flu, or suffer from headaches. It's not just our emotions that feel nurtured by sex. A happy, sexually satisfied body releases all the right hormones and endorphins to keep it looking great as well.

Be a penis genius!
Stuff even he doesn't know about his most precious part

Wanna see some naked breasts? Easy! You'll find just what you're looking for in lots of magazines and movies (and we've not even touched on cable television). Wanna see a naked penis? Sorry. You'll have to hide out in a public restroom for that one. While garden variety, celebrity, and even royal breasts (not to mention toes) are everywhere, not even Joe-average-type penises – let alone the high-profile sort – are regularly caught swaying in the breeze.

When Harvey Kietel appeared full frontal and semierect in *The Piano*, the world gasped. And not just because he's hung like a horse. In most countries and in most conservative mediums, it's illegal to show an erect penis unless it's attached to a Burmese bumblebee on the National Geographic channel. Which is a shame really, since a truly erect, so-hard-it's-going-to-burst, veins-throbbing, blood-pumping penis is a glorious and gladiatorial sight!

You can show a flaccid penis if there's a good – i.e. educational – reason for it. But even men tend to agree that nonerect penises look faintly ridiculous and sort of pointless just dangling there, not really doing anything (like God had a little leftover modeling clay and played a joke on men by rolling it up into a sausage). Hardly surprising, then, that most men aren't jumping up and down saying "Pick me! Pick me!" for the chance to show theirs off in that state. One reason why females are rarely treated to a public sighting.

Men, on the other hand, get plenty of chances to compare their whatnots against everybody else's. Hence the paranoia. If female fears over genitalia aren't helped by the fact that we can't see them without the use of a mirror, men's are probably due to being able to see theirs and other men's equipment in the urinals and common shower-room far too frequently and making too many, often inaccurate, comparisons. (And here's three instantly gratifying reassurances for the truly unnerved before I go any further: 1. A cylindrical object always appears longer and bigger when viewed from the side than when seen from above; 2. Actors in porn films aren't the norm: they're specifically hired because of their abnormally large penis size; 3. The entrance to the vagina – the first third – is more sensitive than the last two-thirds. Further proof that length really doesn't matter. Feeling better already? Fabulous! Now, read on...)

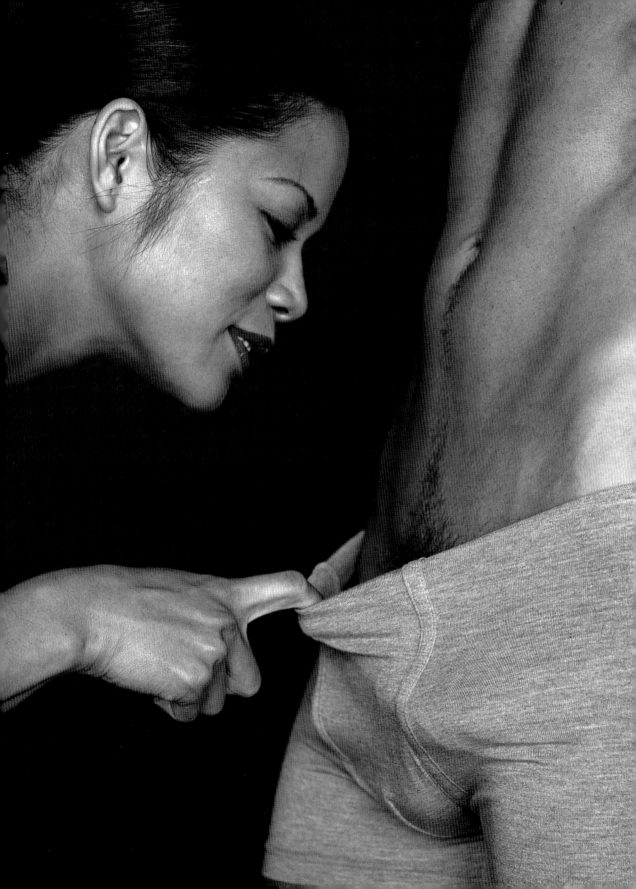

Bernie Zilbergeld (acclaimed sex therapist and author of *The New Male Sexuality*) got it right when he said penis envy does exist…within the male population. While good old (sexist, paranoid, delusional) Sigmund Freud might have coined the term to explain why women are envious of men's dangly parts, the fact is that most aren't (except possibly when desperate to pee outdoors).

Sadly, these days penis envy rings true for a different reason: namely that most men seem to want to trade their penis for someone else's. One which is wider, harder, bigger, longer, and has more staying power than their own. Only one thing stops these men from ever realizing their

Why does one testicle hang lower than the other? It stops them from getting squashed when he walks! Few of our bodies are symmetrical and in 85 percent of males, it's the left that's lower and larger.

FACT 1

MYTH: Bald guys have stronger sex drives.
REALITY: Probably true. The myth says bald men are more virile than men with hair because they have more testosterone in their bodies (which can cause hair loss). The testosterone/hair loss link is true and testosterone is the chemical responsible for his sexual libido.

FACT 2

MYTH: Having sex the night before affects his athletic performance.
REALITY: In a recent study, men who had sex night before a strenuous workout suffered no serious decreases in strength, balance, reaction time, or cardiovascular power the next day. In fact, it might just improve his game because sex relieves pregame stress and tension.

dream of owning the longed-for highly prized deluxe model – and it's not penis transplant surgery. The deluxe model, blessed with all these qualities, only really exists in their imagination. No other part of the male body is more shrouded in myth and folklore than this most precious body part. So, in an attempt to separate fact from fiction, to reassure, and – OK, I admit it – simply to entertain, over these and the next few pages, you'll find a selection of stats and snippets, details and data to sort the fact from the fictitious. Not only will it turn both of you into instant penis geniuses (and make you a huge hit at dinner parties), but it's also guaranteed to make his head swell. In all the right places.

A high testosterone level can get you in trouble. Married men who test above average are more likely to have affairs and (no guesses why) are more likely to end up divorced.

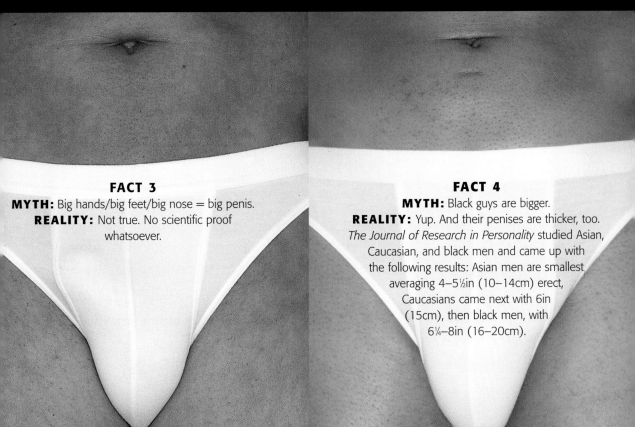

FACT 3
MYTH: Big hands/big feet/big nose = big penis.
REALITY: Not true. No scientific proof whatsoever.

FACT 4
MYTH: Black guys are bigger.
REALITY: Yup. And their penises are thicker, too. *The Journal of Research in Personality* studied Asian, Caucasian, and black men and came up with the following results: Asian men are smallest averaging 4–5½in (10–14cm) erect, Caucasians came next with 6in (15cm), then black men, with 6¼–8in (16–20cm).

STIFF COMPETITION

- Despite differences when flaccid, most erect penises are around the same size. (Some penises actually double in length.)
- Average erect size range: 5–6 inches (13–15cm). Flaccid size range: 2–4 inches (5–10cm).
- Smallest functional penis recorded on a man: ⅞ inch (1.8cm).
- Largest functional penis recorded on a man: 11 inches (28cm).
- Average increase after penile enlargement surgery: flaccid, 3 inches (7.6cm); erect, 1inch (2.5cm).
- Amount of blood in a flaccid penis: 3oz (9ml); amount in erect penis: 30oz (90ml).
- Around 60 percent of men in the US are circumcised, compared with an international average of 23 percent. Rates of circumcision have declined in the US since a peak of 85 percent in 1980.
- Men with large testicles are more likely to cheat on their partners and to have 30 percent more sex than men with smaller testicles. (Levels of testosterone are higher in men with larger testicles.)

There's more protein in an average ejaculation than a medium-sized pork chop.
Choose to swallow rather than spit and you've provided your body with a large part of your daily dose of protein!

GOING UP?

- The average time a man can keep an erection: 40 minutes. The younger the man, the longer he can keep it up.
- Average speed of ejaculation: 28mph (45kph).
- Percentage of men who say they climax too early: 30.
- Average number of erections per day for a man: 7. Average number of erections that occur while he's asleep: 5.
- The penis has a safety valve to ensure that a man can't ejaculate and urinate at the same time.
- Only one-third of impotency cases are due to physical problems. Ninety percent are treatable.

TRIVIAL PURSUITS

- According to researchers at Taiwan University, waiting too long to urinate can reduce blood flow to your heart by about 25 percent.
- Two in every thousand men are capable of giving themselves fellatio.
- The tissue that surrounds the penis is more durable than the tissue that surrounds the brain.
- Distance sperm travels to fertilize an egg: 3–4 inches (7.5–10cm). Human equivalent: 26 miles.

Ball games

- Testicles disappear when a man gets cold or as he approaches orgasm. It's a reflex action. They retract into his body during intercourse as a protective instinct, so they don't get knocked around. Testes also produce and care for semen, which must be kept at a constant temperature (lower than the rest of the body but not freezing), so testicles rise and fall against the body depending on how much heat they need. Hence all the hype about tight jeans, which hold the testes too close to the body, making men infertile. This is why the testes are stored away from the body in their own little custom-made carrier, the scrotum.

- Does the size of testicles indicate fertility? Larger testicles produce more sperm but size doesn't affect quality. To produce vigorous sperm quit smoking, cut back on alcohol, exercise regularly, and eat well. That's right: the more boring (aka healthy) you are, the more likely you are to become a dad. (Consider it future training for all those nights in once the little treasure arrives.)

- The largest testicles in the world belong to…your boyfriend. Nope. Wrong answer. It's the Northern White Whale, which wins the prize with testicles that can weigh up to 2,200lbs (990 kilograms).

- The testes also produce the male sex hormone, testosterone. Testosterone levels peak early morning, which is – gosh! what a surprise! – when most men want sex the most.

- Zinc supplements or normal exercise increase supplies of testosterone. Stress or exhaustive exercise decrease it. When levels run low, men are irritable, depressed, and sleepy.

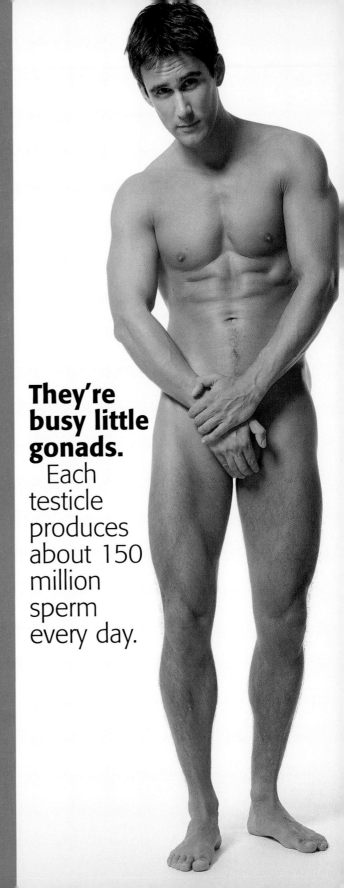

They're busy little gonads. Each testicle produces about 150 million sperm every day.

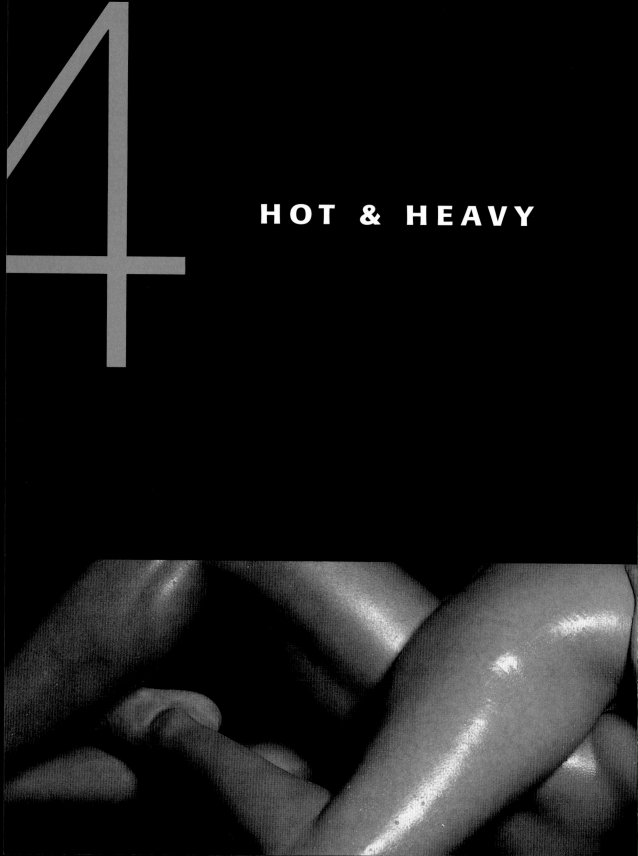

4

HOT & HEAVY

Delve into the **murky depths** of the male mind. Find tips to turn you into the best lover she's ever had, **show-off sex** positions you'll *both* **adore,** and instant fix-its to send your sex life soaring.

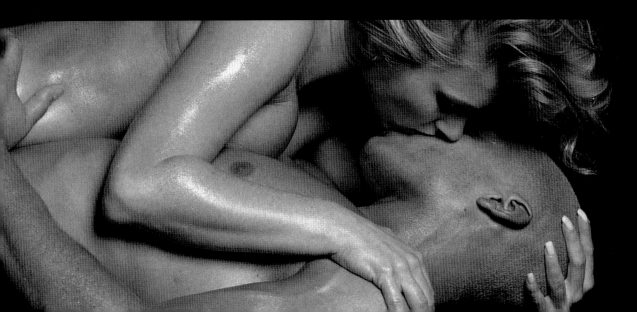

16

Sex tricks
to instantly transform your love life

Great sex does take time – but that's not to say there aren't plenty of little tricks that'll get you there faster! I asked 20 couples, all of whom described themselves as "above average" lovers, to test out the following techniques, which are designed to give an instant zap to your sex life. They rated them for enjoyment, and I took an average to give you a raunch rating. (Of course, to be absolutely sure my math is correct, it's probably a very good idea for you to personally test each and every one of them yourselves…)

GIVE A HAND-JOB

1 For a different type of hand-job (but one that's equally as delicious) try the following:
For him Make him squirm in public by sucking his finger as though it's a small penis. Lean forward so no one else can see you (if you've got long hair, hide behind it), maintain eye contact, hold his finger in your mouth, and swirl and lick and suck until he can't take it any longer. Unless you're lavishly licking up and down his finger like it's a lollipop, it's relatively easy to get away with it without being arrested. In other words, keep most of the action happening inside your mouth (even if there is a lot happening in his jeans).
For her Return the public humiliation by lifting her hand to your mouth as though you're going to kiss the back of it, then turning it over and burying your tongue in her palm. As with the above, do like you'd do if you were giving her oral sex. Again, if you hold her hand at the right angle and keep most of the tongue action close, Aunt Betty could be watching and simply think you're being romantic. Well, she will until your girlfriend literally slides off her chair.

VIBRATE WITH PLEASURE

Don't leave it shoved in the back of a drawer, rescued only when he's gone to a baseball game and you've got the house to yourself! Vibrators are the zero-effort, quick, and convenient way to orgasm if you're both tired or don't have much time.

For him Apply it to knotted, aching shoulders and the cheeks of his bottom before moving down to concentrate on the perineum – the area between his anus and testicles. Let him get used to the feeling before trying it out (on a low speed) on his testicles (cup them in one hand) and the opening of his anus. Depending on what sort of vibrator you have, you might like to insert it inside his rectum (definitely ask if the idea appeals first, though, and use tons of lubricant!), while giving him oral sex or masturbating him with your hands.

RAUNCHRATING **6/10**

For her Again, use it on her shoulders, back, and feet, before moving to the obvious. Contrary to what the porn industry would have us believe, most women don't insert vibrators, but hold them firmly against the closed labia, sometimes massaging in small circles or using a press-then-lift motion, while applying varying pressure. She knows how she likes it, so it's a good idea to let her show you how it's done. After that, it's a weapon in your hands as you buzz, tease, and take her right to the brink…then back again (and again). Vibrators are terrific if she's horny and you're not, or if you both want an orgasm but don't have the time or energy for anything that requires effort.

RAUNCHRATING **9/10**

TELL A BEDTIME STORY

Forget Harry Potter, think Harry Does Sally.

For him Make up your own erotic tale or borrow one of his old girlie mags and use a story from the back. Lead him into the bedroom, tuck him into bed, sit by the bed on a chair, and open a book (any will do, it's being used as a prop only). Then proceed to tell him the dirtiest, sexiest, most erotic fantasy scenario you can bear to say out loud. He's allowed to touch himself but not you. Let him masturbate himself to orgasm as you reach the climax of your tale.

RAUNCHRATING **8/10**

For her Indulge a popular female fantasy: sex with a stranger. Blindfold her. Tie her hands behind her back. Lead her into a dark room and leave her standing alone for a few minutes. Then enter the room stealthily, come up behind her, and tell her you're the handsome stranger who's admired her from afar. She has a boyfriend but she's arranged to meet you, her unknown admirer, in a hotel room.

RAUNCHRATING **9/10**

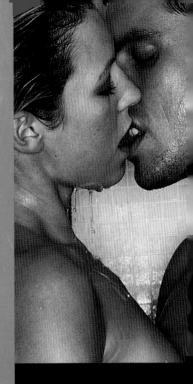

Vibrators are terrific if **she's horny** and you're not, or if you **both want an orgasm** but don't have the time or energy for anything that requires effort.

TURN OFF THE LIGHTS

For both of you After years of working up to having sex with all the lights on (yes, it takes most men that long to convince us they're not looking at the cellulite on our thighs or our wobbly tummies), I'm now suggesting you not only turn the lights off but make the room as close to total darkness as possible. Then blindfold each other. Why? By removing the sense of sight, you heighten all others – most particularly touch. (It's the reason why lots of people close their eyes while kissing or during sex, so they can focus fully on the sensation.) Robbed of our eyesight, we're also more aware of each other's breathing and moaning, and all the other sounds of sex, which tend to get lost when we can see. Yet another bonus: there's an element of surprise. Once your lover breaks contact, you can't see where they're headed next, until you feel a hand caressing the inside of your thigh, hear some shockingly filthy thoughts whispered in your ear, and feel a tongue in the place you least expected it.

RAUNCHRATING RAUNCHRATING **8/10** RAUNCHRATING RAUNCHRATING

Robbed of our eyesight, we're also more aware of each other's **breathing and moaning** and all the other **sounds of sex,** which tend to get lost when we can see.

HAVE A TONGUE TUSSLE

Did you honestly think I could write this without including some type of oral sex tip? Shame on you! While I could go on for hours about tongue technique for both of you (and I do – see The definitive guide to oral sex, pp.60–67), it does happen to be the most important part of it all. Practice makes perfect, and if you get this part right, the rest pales in comparison.

For him Concentrate your tongue action on the frenulum (the stringy part at the head of the penis on the underside, where the head meets the shaft). While your mouth is closed around his penis creating a warm, firm vacuum, make s-l-o-w circles around the rim of the head, giving a double lick and wiggle every time you pass the frenulum. Don't do it for too long if you're planning on intercourse afterward – he won't last that long!

For her Instantly improve the most inexperienced oral sex technique by using the whole flat area of your tongue, rather than just the tip. Forget what you see in the porn movies – they tense their tongues and stick them out so you see more action. Reality is different. Try it on your own palm and you'll see what I mean. First use the tip of your tongue to lick your palm. Note how it only stimulates

RAUNCHRATING RAUNCHRATING **8/10** RAUNCHRATING RAUNCHRATING a tiny area and can be quite rough. Now lay the whole top surface of your tongue flat against your palm. It covers a much larger area of skin and feels wetter, gentler, and softer. She's not the only one who'll benefit: your tongue is far less likely to get tired using it flat rather than pointed, because it's relaxed, not tensed. A flat tongue works much better on your testicles too.

CREATE A FANTASY

For both of you Hate mobile phones and computers? Bet you won't after this! Keep things steamy when you're apart by emailing or texting the first two sentences of a steamy fantasy, along with an instruction for them to send it back with the next two sentences added. Not only does it make that commute home a whole lot more interesting, but it's also a great way of coming up with fantasies that appeal to both of you, since both of you have equal input into what happens. Keep going back and forth with the game until you both come home to…turn it into reality, of course!

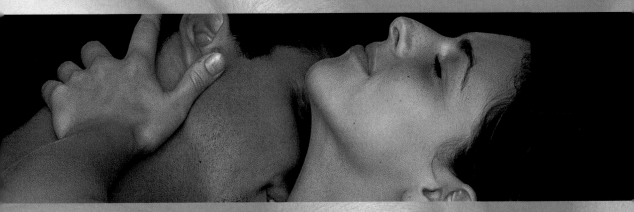

DRIVE HIM NUTS

For him Get ballsy by taking control of his. It is a matter of personal preference – some men hate having their testicles stimulated, while others love it – but it's worth trying. So often they're left shyly hanging back there, while the star of the show, his penis, gets all the attention and affection. Be a fan, perfect your ballgame, and you hold the key to his sexual heaven in your hot little hands. Think of his testicles in the same way he thinks of your breasts. You can cradle them, suck them, stroke them, knead them. What you can't and shouldn't do, though, is bite or pull them too hard. They're sensitive all over but take a closer look the next time you're giving him oral. Search for a little ridge running up the middle, then follow it until you find the piece of skin that joins his testicles to his penis. This is usually the most sensitive part. It's best stimulated with your tongue but use lubricant or your fingers (and saliva) and trace the area with your fingertips. Also try circling the area where testicles and penis meet with the tip of your tongue, flicking it back and forth. Or use your tongue to lick swirling patterns around each testicle. Later, when you've started fellating him, you can use one hand to lightly cup his testicles and gently "juggle" them.

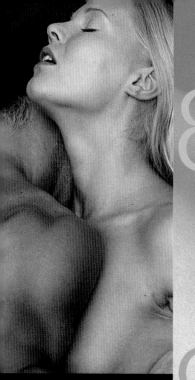

The bed picnic is **infinitely versatile…** (birthdays, Valentine's Day… Tuesday nights **when there's nothing on the TV).**

TURN IT UPSIDE DOWN

For both of you The upside-down 69er was invented by Alex Comfort (Mr. *Joy of Sex*) and it's never been bettered! She lies sideways across the bed and lowers her body to the floor, almost as though she's doing a handstand. Her head and palms rest on the floor; her legs and torso are still on the bed. He kneels on the bed in between her legs. Because she's upside down, the pressure in the veins of the face and neck produce quite startling sensations. Don't like it? Then let yourself be tempted by some tantric: "The Crow" is the rather exotic name for the classic 69er position turned on its side: you both lie on your sides, head to toe, facing each other. Each of you draws your inner thigh up so it can be used as a cushion for your partner's head. It's a simple variation on the norm but a lot more comfortable for both of you.

RAUNCHRATING RAUNCHRATING RAUNCHRATING RAUNCHRATING **8** /10

STARTLE THE SENSES

For both of you They do it in the movies but few of us use ice cubes anywhere but in drinks. Shame really, because an ice cold mouth pressed against hot genitals feels exquisite! Put a glass full of small ice cubes nearby when you're having sex and pop some in your mouth before you fellate him; insert one into her vagina before performing oral sex (a very small cube – you want to chill not numb). If ice cubes feel too startling, try chilled champagne, ice cream, or chilled, creamy yogurt instead. Next, raise the temperature all around by adding a hot drink and alternating the two sensations. Follow a few minutes of stimulation with a cool mouth by a few minutes of stimulation by a hot mouth. By varying temperature and taste, you're activating two sets of nerve endings to serve up a sensory smorgasbord.

RAUNCHRATING RAUNCHRATING RAUNCHRATING RAUNCHRATING **9** /10

COUNTDOWN TO ECSTASY

For him Are you finding it's all over a little faster than you'd both like? Count backwards from 500 while having intercourse. Your brain's kept busy, so your penis is also distracted. Zero is blast off! Another technique, courtesy of Carole Altman, enables you to isolate awareness of swelling in the penis and testicles and the movement of fluid. Do each step over one week: 1. Masturbate slowly, stopping as soon as you feel yourself getting erect; 2. Stroke until you get a slight erection, but go one or two strokes further; 3. Stroke but pay attention to feelings in the testicles. The minute you feel tightening and lifting, stop; 4. Stroke until conscious of testicle sensations, then try one or two strokes further; 5. Stroke until aware of the flow of semen in your penis, then with your thumb press hard on the vein running along the outside of the penis head.

RAUNCHRATING RAUNCHRATING RAUNCHRATING RAUNCHRATING **8** /10

11

PLAN A BED PICNIC

For her You need: champagne on ice, food you can eat with your fingers (chocolates, exotic canapés) and food you can smear all over each other (honey, ice cream, cream, yogurt). Mobile phones off, telly and video moved to a prime position, and all that's left to do is slide an erotic movie into the video and settle in. The bed picnic's infinitely versatile and suitable for all sorts of occasions (birthdays, Valentine's Day, Tuesday nights when there's nothing on TV…). Vary it by replacing the naughty video with some sex books. Go to any good bookstore and grab an armful that cover the areas that particularly tickle your fancy (tantric, how to tantalize your lover while wearing galoshes, how to have a dozen orgasms in five minutes flat – whatever does it for you). You don't have to read them cover to cover, just skim them for inspiration on how to keep things fresh and imaginative. Earmark the pages that cover the things you want to try; find the good parts and read them aloud to each other as foreplay. It's also a great way to get you both talking openly about sex. If you're not terribly good at expressing yourself, it's much easier and less embarrassing to point to something and say "That looks great – I'd love it if you did that to me" than it is to say "I'd really like you to get on all fours and make like a horse so I can ride you."

RAUNCH RATING 7/10

12

TAKE A DETOUR

For him Can't have penetrative sex because you've got a UTI/your period? Have "pretend" vaginal sex by lubricating his penis, keeping your thighs firmly together, and letting him thrust between them. Position yourself so his penis is sliding through the lips of your vagina, stimulating the clitoris, but no penetration is allowed. You can try this standing up, lying down, or from behind. Alternatively, try gluteal sex (from gluteus, the muscles of the buttocks): he applies lots of lubricant to his penis, you lie on your stomach and put a pillow under your hips. He then thrusts between the cheeks of your buttocks. Or oil your breasts and hold them firmly together, while he thrusts in between.

RAUNCH RATING 7/10

13

PLAY MIND GAMES

For him Play the primitive. Lure him into the bedroom where he'll find you lying flat on your tummy with your bottom in the air. Completely bare your genitals when he least expects it, this is real monkey-in-the-zoo stuff. Women don't usually do it because it makes them feel vulnerable, but if you know him well and trust him, why not? I'm not saying it doesn't go against everything she's ever been taught (it's not ladylike/it's crude/hardly playing hard to get/the complete opposite of "coy," not-at-all nice girl), but quite frankly, all the more reason to do it.

RAUNCH RATING 6/10

For her Ask her which actor she'd most like to take to bed, then make up a fantasy for her. Tape record it for her, so she can masturbate to it when you're not around. As you're having sex, repeat it out loud, acting it out as you go. (There's no need to be jealous – it's highly unlikely she'll get the opportunity to do the same with Brad Pitt in real life.) A birthday treat that beats the hell out of flowers? Ask her to write down her top 10 turn-ons and deliver one a day for the next 10 days. Time the first or last to coincide with the birthday.

RAUNCH RATING 6/10

BE A SEX SLAVE

For both of you Be their sex slave for a day – yup, that's one entire day devoted to pleasuring them! They get to order you around – and whether it's making the bed or making whoopee, you're not allowed to utter even ONE word of complaint. Up the anticipatory factor by sending a card in the mail with the message "On (whatever date) I will be your sex slave for the entire day. Do with me what you will." That gives them plenty of time to think about what they're going to do with the time. Add three questions at the end: What do you want me to wear? (do you need to buy anything to fulfill the fantasy?); Anything you crave, besides me? (food, alcohol); Anything else I need to make your dreams come true? (props if you're role-playing a fantasy). They don't need to forewarn you of what they've got planned (that would ruin the surprise), but the more they've thought about it, the better. Nothing worse than having psyched yourself up into subservience, presented yourself as a slave and your partner goes bright red, shuffles their feet, and then says "Er, um, what would *you* like to do?"

14

RAUNCHRATING RAUNCHRATING RAUNCHRATING RAUNCHRATING **8/10**

Bury your tongue in her palm, doing as you'd do if you were giving her oral sex. **Aunt Betty** will simply think you're being romantic…Well, she will until your girlfriend literally **slides off her chair.**

MIX IT UP A BIT

For both of you I'm a huge fan of take-turns sex. Instead of both of you trying to give and receive, take turns at being "the giver" and "the taker" and stop feeling guilty. It's incredibly hard, for instance, to really enjoy the sensation of someone giving you oral sex – no matter how fabulous they are at it – if you're also concentrating on using your hand to masturbate them at the same time. Well, next time don't! Let them concentrate exclusively on you. The thing is, no matter how multi-dexterous you are, few of us do a great job of it anyway because we're much more interested in what's being done to us. Selfish little sausages that we (all) are. (This is one reason why I think 69ers are completely overrated. The concept's nice but, in reality, you're both fixated on your own pleasure.) While we're on the topic of mixing things up, vary the style of sex you have as well. Ideally, you'd enjoy a mix of bread-and-butter sex (you just get it over with because you're both tired and have to be up early for meetings); adventurous sex ("naughty" stuff where lust overtakes or you plan and try out new things); he sex (sex that focuses mainly on him); she sex (sex that focuses mainly on her); and a healthy smattering of quickie sex (sometimes because you're hot

15

and bothered, other times because time or energy is restricted). Take an average of how many sex sessions you'd have per month, then decide together how you'd like to distribute them. Take into account what's realistic given life pressures, but be a little aspirational!

RAUNCHRATING 10/10

GO ON A PLEASURE HUNT

For him Get your best friend to take some sexy pictures of you naked (use a Polaroid camera or the man at the drugstore is never going to look at you the same way again). Get her to photograph you in all sorts of erotic poses (the more explicit, the sexier it is, but you might want to point and aim the camera yourself for the really naughty up-close ones. For example, your friend might know you've got a Brazilian wax but it's unlikely she wants to see it in that much detail). The trick is to use a combination of arty/flattering/erotic poses: aim for one-third of the photos to be the sort a traditional (if slightly risqué) photographer would take; one third to be the sort of glam shots you'd see in the girlie magazines; the remaining should be make-your-grandmother's-eyes-water, all-out porn

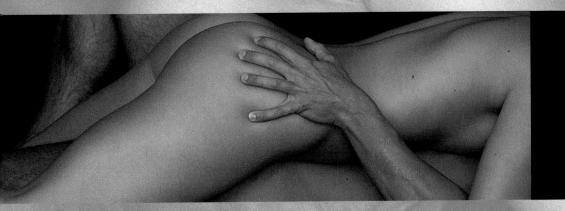

photofeasts. A lethal combination of sensual/sexy/slam-right-between-the-eyeballs! Once you've finished composing your erotic masterpieces, stop by the supermarket for a big box of chocolates (choose ones that come separately wrapped), then head straight back home to make yourself gorgeous. Pour a glass of wine to steady your nerves, pour yourself into the sexiest lingerie you own, then make a trail of chocolates to lure your prey into the ultimate honey-trap. Place a note ("You're on a pleasure hunt. Follow the chocolates…"), the tamest photograph and the first chocolate where he can't possibly miss them after walking in the door. Then strategically place each photograph between there and your hideout, the photos getting saucier the closer he gets, all linked up by the chocolates. By the time he's devoured the visual feast, he should arrive at the door, frothing and foaming at the mouth with anticipation, to find you provocatively posed and beautifully lit by candles strategically placed by the bed. If, instead, he enters with only chocolate smears, he's either 1. Hypoglycemic and desperate for a sugar fix; 2. Just come back from having sex with his mistress; Or 3. been tampered with by aliens, who have sucked all the testosterone from his body. In all cases except 1, put clothes back on.

RAUNCHRATING 9/10

What he wants you to do more of...
Venturing into the murky depths of the male mind

Here's where we explore the dirty – some might say downright filthy – side of the male psyche to find out what really makes him tick. Now, lots of you will be tempted to skip over this part in an attempt to ignore the less savory side of his sexuality. Please don't. This is the stuff you'd hear if you bugged your guy's beer glass, so you just might learn something. Forewarned is forearmed, and besides – it's not that bad! I've written this section assuming that it will be read mainly by women, but I've also added some "Sneak tips for him." These are for men hoping to pick up tips on how to persuade her to be more adventurous. I'm not implying for a moment that all the stuff here doesn't apply to women as well as men, but you have to generalize at some point to make sense of the world (and a book).

FACT 1: MEN LIKE NAUGHTY THINGS

First, let's define "naughty." The liberated among you will already be thinking things like: slightly kinky, forbidden, racy, i.e. healthy, thoughts. Others might not. In society, there's a clear line drawn between "normal" and "naughty," between what's accepted and what's not. The definition appears to be this: if everyone does it, no matter what "it" is, it's "normal" and therefore OK to admit to. If only a few do it, no matter what "it" is, it becomes "sick" or "weird." Sorry, but I'm with US sexpert Carole Altman and others worldwide who say that if you want to march to the music of a different drum, why not? As she says, so long as you're not stomping on someone else or kicking yourself in the process, what's the problem? The moral: try really hard not to have a knee-jerk reaction if your partner suggests something unusual. Think first: Does what he wants hurt anyone, physically or emotionally? Is there any danger? Then what's the problem? Be one of the few women to embrace this concept and you'll never be alone on a date night again (unless you want to be). Add an understanding of how much men's sexual arousal is dependent on what they see and you'll have them lining up around the block. Visual excitement is his number one turn-on. Evidence the many letters I get on the topic: Why won't she… watch porn/shave off her pubes/wear sexy clothes/leave her shoes on/watch in a mirror/masturbate for me/go out without underwear? What he is saying is that he wants something he's not used to seeing or doing. As with most things, it all comes down to variety, but it's not that difficult to serve up a different treat each time. Think hamburgers. (Yes, really.) One night he gets his hamburger with cheese. The next cheese and bacon. Then chili. Then maybe pickles…you get the picture.

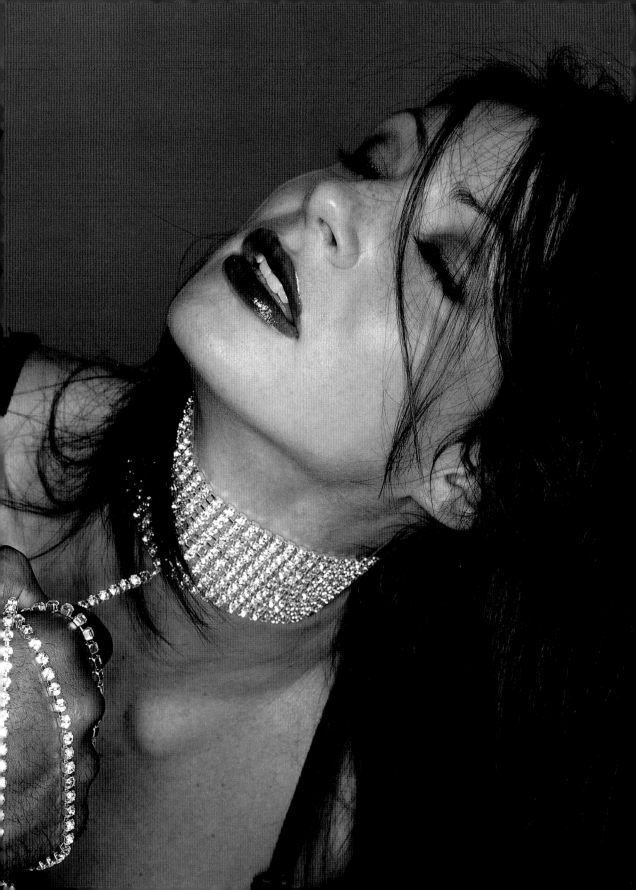

Some women find the male addiction to variety and gadgets/situations threatening. Why? Because there's a dark side to male sexuality that operates on an intrinsically primitive level. Unleash it and you can't help but see evidence of raw, uncontrollable emotion. I think it's the "uncontrollable" aspect that worries women. It's a little frightening. We think, "If he loves doing it this much, what hope do I have of him being faithful if I say no or he stops wanting me?" Admittedly, the stats aren't great: about 50 percent of men are unfaithful. But women are fast becoming just as untrustworthy, and if you make it clear he can ask *you* for the "kinky" stuff, he won't have to go to someone else for it, will he?

It takes him back to the heady experience of (gasp) **getting his hand inside** his girlfriend's top or (double gasp) **her panties.**

FACT 2: MEN LIKE HAVING SEX IN FORBIDDEN PLACES

Sex in unusual, risky, and semipublic places rates high on most men's wish lists. Hence, why he's always hassling you to have a quickie in the bathroom at parties, in the toilet on planes, in your parents' bedroom (have you noticed, never in his?) and – how could we forget? – the most popular sex request: being given oral sex while cruising along the highway. Men like sex in cars. It takes him back to adolescent fumblings and the heady experience of (gasp) getting his hand inside his girlfriend's top or (double gasp) her panties. Back then, sex was not only forbidden (and therefore naughtier) but simple. There's only so much you can get up to in a car because of space limitations, so even the simplest act becomes erotic – which means the pressure's off. Throw in an element of exhibitionism and you can see why he loves it.

A little harder to come to grips with: him wanting to do it in places like public restrooms. Yes, it has gay connotations and it sounds (and probably is) unhygienic. But that's the point. It's sex stripped of its niceties and brought back to the basics: hot flesh against cold concrete. The fact that the ultragroomed George Michael was willing to risk lots of bad publicity for sex in a public restroom speaks volumes.

Sneak tip for him: talk her into it by…
Telling her she's great in bed. The sexier she feels and the better she thinks she is at sex, the more inclined she'll be to try new things. You won't get anywhere by telling her your other girlfriends didn't have a problem with it/she's boring/unimaginative. All that does is strip her of her self-confidence and make her even less inclined to go outside her comfort zone. Trying to push her into doing something by nagging also backfires. The more you nag, the more determined she'll be to hold out. It becomes a war of wills. The secret to talking her into doing anything she's nervous about? Send a very clear message: *I want you more than I want to do this.* Followed closely by: *you don't have to agree if you don't want to.*

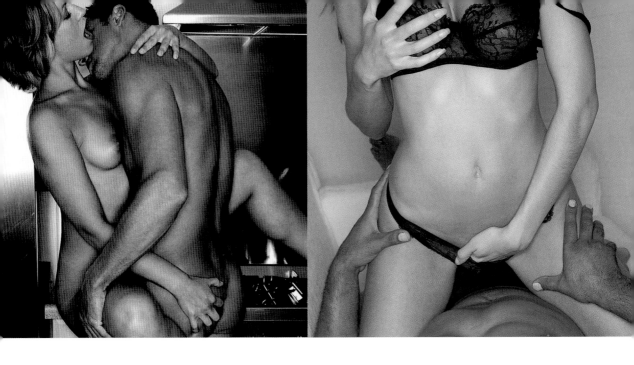

FACT 3: MEN LIKE LOOKING AT NAUGHTY THINGS

Let's get straight to it, shall we? Pubic hair. What's his opinion on what to do about it? Should you leave it as it is, trim it, or wax all of it off with the flick of a beautician's fair hand? It's a matter of taste really. Some women leave their pubic hair *au naturel* and some men love it like that. But I'd say the majority of us give it a trim and shave or wax the "bikini line" (hair which protrudes past our panties or bikini bottom) and the majority of men put their hands up to vote "Yes! good idea." A minority shave it all off (beyond itchy when it's growing back) and an increasing number brave a Brazilian wax (removal of all hair from the genitals and anus by wax). I use the word "brave" not just because it hurts like hell but because it involves getting on very intimate terms with a beauty therapist by either kneeling on all fours and sticking your butt high in the air or lying down and trying to put your feet behind your ears. Not for the shy or inflexible! Some women worry that a partner who prefers women who remove their pubic hair has a tendency toward pedophilia (because the smooth, hairless appearance resembles the genitals of children). There are no facts or research to support this, and the majority of men who want you bald request it because it's something new/it's a little kinky/it makes oral sex easier. So quit worrying about that and focus your paranoia on something far more likely to come true: ingrown hairs. All bikini waxers fear them more than the scales. They sound harmless enough but the end result is horrible purplish lumps that look awful and take ages to go away. Not a good look.

OK, now that we've got that out of the way, let's add a few more things – like clothes. It's ironic really: we think men spend all their time undressing us with their eyes and, in fact, the opposite is often happening. They're adding a G-string, a push-up bra, a pair of stilettos, a rubber dress. This is one area where most women will indulge him. Those who won't, worry (mostly unnecessarily) that it will turn into a fetish. Which is why my advice to him on this would be to wait awhile…

Sneak tip for him: talk her into it by…

Asking her in the right way. There's an enormous difference between telling a girl you've just met that you have a thing for shoes (and would she mind awfully if she left hers on) and waiting for the relationship and trust to develop, then saying "Wow! You'd look great in those!" after spying some suitable skyscrapers. All you need to do is buy her an impromptu gift of shoes, get her to model them, and – Gosh! How did that happen? – leave them on during the sex which follows. The first scenario reeks of dirty old man and sex for sex's sake; the second works because she already knows you find her sexy with the shoes off. It's not about the shoes, it's about HER wearing them. Get it? Make it very clear it's still *her* you're making love to, not the object.

There's a dark side to **male sexuality** that operates on an **intrinsically primitive level.** Unleash it and you can't help but see evidence of **raw, uncontrollable emotion.**

FACT 4: MEN LIKE DOING NAUGHTY THINGS

Men like doing new things. So do women, dogs, cats, and probably lampposts, if they could articulate the thought (at least we get to move around). Which is why, when he says something like "I wish you'd do more to me in bed," it makes us angry. Like 1. Hello! Don't you think I'd like something more original than two quick grabs of the breasts, then your hand sliding…? 2. It sounds like criticism, and 3. A lot like a demand as well ("You're not doing enough! Do more!"). No wonder we end up feeling resentful. And there's another reason why we're not rushing to pull on that Batgirl suit/try position no. 645/wear garters and stockings: the embarrassment factor. Looking fat or feeling ridiculous is the main reason women cite for not being more adventurous. It has a lot to do with timing as well. "Can I tie you up?" said with the right attitude/timing/expression/intonation could be the best thing we've heard since "Prada is having a shoe sale." Choose the wrong moment, wrong tone, and wrong time and forget it.

Sneak tip for him: talk her into it by…

Coming at it from a position of strength. "I love everything you do to me in bed." Not only is it a compliment, but it also gives her permission to fail (she can do no wrong so isn't scared to make a fool of herself). Reassure her that you're just as likely to feel embarrassed/silly or burst out laughing and that you'll be laughing with her, not at her, if all goes wrong. It's often simply a matter of giving her – actually make that both of you – permission not just to laugh, but really laugh, if things go horribly wrong. Just in case you haven't gotten the message, it's OK to laugh as well as lust, besides, better to laugh than be over-serious. Which is why if you are suggesting tie-up games, use a scarf or her stockings, not something scary like rope or string. Fear and excitement are two sides of the same coin, and the idea is to get the right balance.

The bottom line

Yes, I am talking bottom line as in…well, bottoms. I know, it's a delicate topic (and feel free to avert your eyes, though God knows how you're supposed to do that and read at the same time). But this delicate topic is getting more and more popular, and there's not much information out there about bottom sex so I'm going for it. Bottoms are an intensely private zone as in "Halt! Who goes there?" i.e. you need permission to enter. So if you're planning on exploring his, either ask outright or read body language: ideally both. Instigate proceedings by stroking the perineum (the smooth area between the anus and testes), then use three fingers and massage firmly. Let your fingers casually brush against his anus and see how he reacts. If he pulls away or clenches his cheeks together, then he's either not interested or he's nervous (possibly both). If he lifts his butt or presses against your hand, it's a pretty good indication that he'd like you to continue, but even so, I'd still say something like "Can I go there?" (even the most embarrassed can usually squeak out "Yes" or "Mmm…"). Before you do, apply some lubricant to your finger and around the whole anal area. Continue stroking the opening until he's relaxed again, then insert the tip of a finger into his rectum. Hold still for a moment or two, then try circling or moving your finger gently in and out. Check that all is fine (just say "OK?") before pushing your finger further inside. Once you've gently explored how deep and what sort of movement he likes, you can add it to oral sex or when you're masturbating him with your hands, just before he's about to orgasm. (For more on anal intercourse, see p.107.)

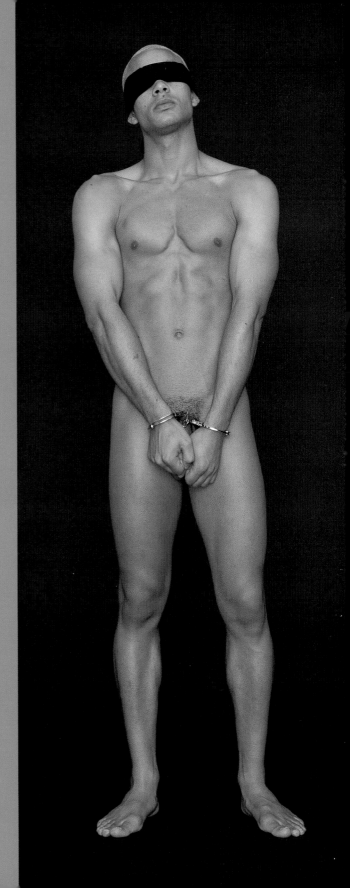

FACT 5: MEN LIKE PLAYING NAUGHTY GAMES

- **Wait on him like Grandma did for Grandad** Greet him after a hard day at the office with a huge hug. Put a drink in his hand. Warm his slippers by the fire. Serve him comfort food for dinner. Give him a shoulder massage while he watches what he wants on TV. Then – and this is crucial – he gets to drift off to sleep with NO SEX. You want him nice and rested to fully appreciate what's on the following night's agenda. Which is…

- **A full body massage with oil and fluffy towels** You dressed in high heels, a G-string, and nothing else (or sexy panties and push-up bra if you prefer – the high heels aren't optional). You can touch him, but he can't touch you. Again, while you tease him by touching his genitals, don't let him climax. No other sexual contact – or release – until day three when you treat him to…

- **A two-hour sex session where you take control** He lies back while you instigate everything and do all the work. Start by stroking him all over, follow with the best oral sex he's ever received (stopping before he gets too excited), then put the poor guy out of his misery by climbing on top.

It's ironic: we think men spend all their time **undressing us with their eyes** and, in fact, the **opposite is often happening**…

- **Completely make his day by suggesting a masturbating competition** The first person to finish (i.e. orgasm) wins the prize (make it good). Cheat by putting on such an award-winning performance, he can't help but let go first just by watching you.

FACT 6: MEN WISH WOMEN WERE AS NAUGHTY AS THEY WERE

Can a woman let loose and play it like the guys do? Probably the most honest answer I can come up with is yes – but only for a little while. Lots of women enjoy sex for sex's sake. Plenty relish the odd flingette. But if that's all they're doing – continually on the hunt for one-night-stands – I don't think too many women would be satisfied long-term. Women seem to tire of singles sex more quickly than men do – and there could be a scientific reason for it. A recent university study found that there's a hormone created in the female after intercourse that helps her form a bond with her partner. Oxytocin, produced by the pituitary gland, also appears to be involved in creating a bond between mother and child as it is also released during breast-feeding. Apparently, the more sex a woman has with the same partner, the more oxytocin is produced, which deepens the bond – on her side, at least.

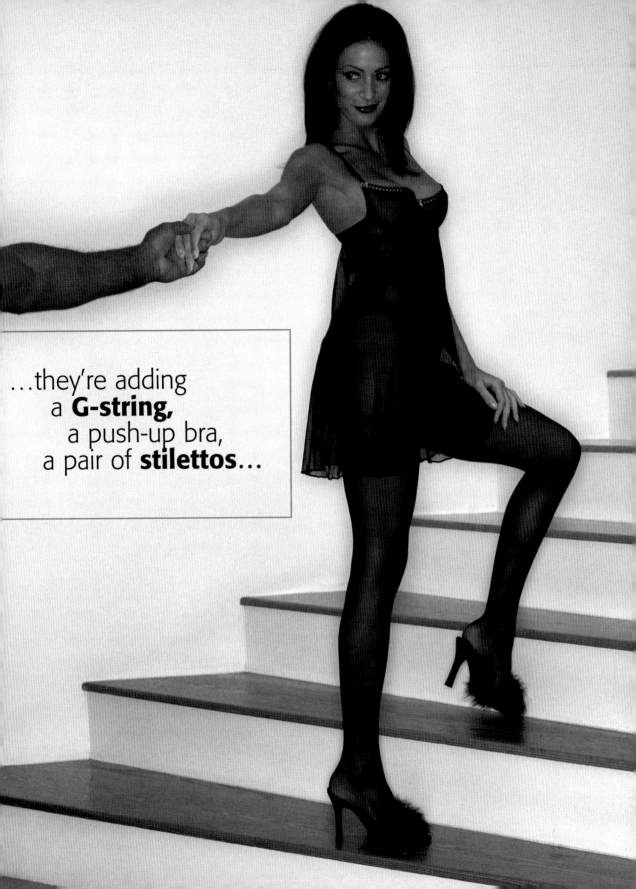

…they're adding
a **G-string,**
a push-up bra,
a pair of **stilettos**…

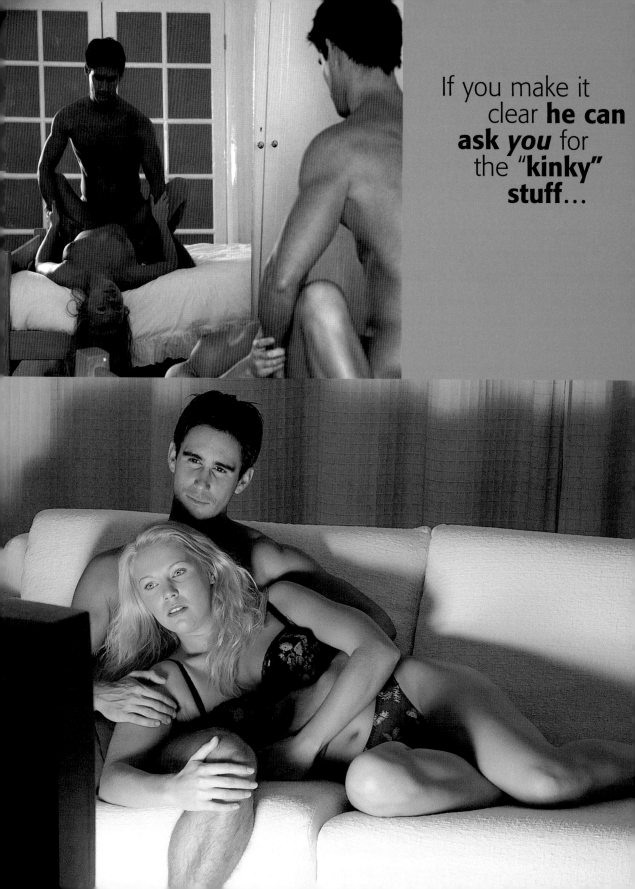

If you make it
clear **he can
ask *you*** for
the "**kinky**"
stuff…

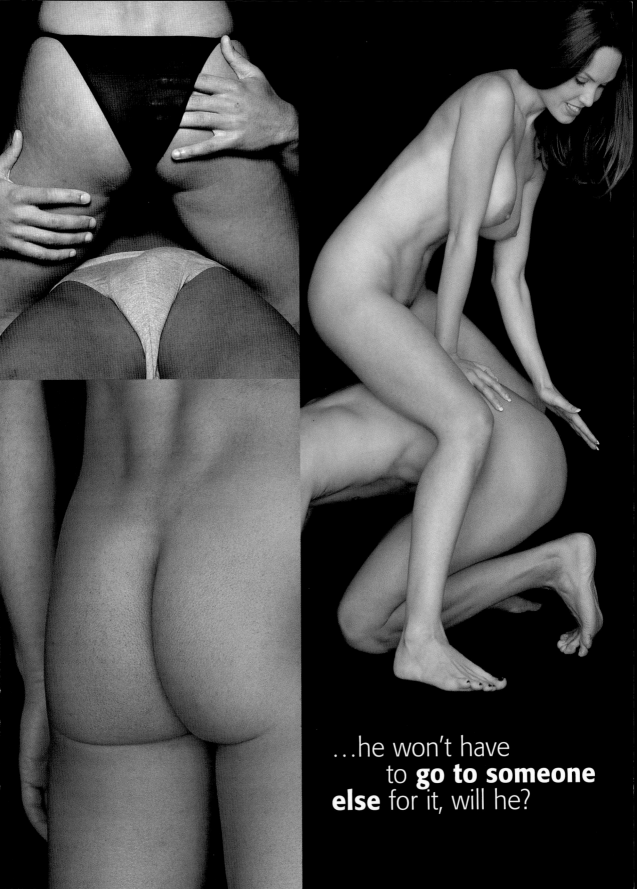

…he won't have to **go to someone else** for it, will he?

10

Guaranteed turn-ons
to make you the best lover she's ever had

Great lovers aren't born, they're made. The more you know about what turns her on, the better lover you'll be. Assuming your girlfriend's not the type that demands freshly blow-dried fluffy white kittens in the bedroom before she'll let you even touch her, each of these 10 tips should elevate you to superlover status pretty rapidly. (If you are hooked up with a fluffy type, you're on your own.) Anyway, here it is: all the stuff that normally only gets spilled – along with the wine – on those girls' nights out.

1 SIT STILL AND LISTEN

Men bond through action, by doing things for women. Women bond with words. Fact: if you want great sex, you're going to have to talk to her – even more important is that you listen. I know your eyes are glazing over already (and I promise this won't all be about burning candles and rearranging your bedroom so it's all feng-shuified). But this part's important to us, and (here's two carrots) not only will it pay off big time in the bedroom (the more listened-to she feels, the more likely she is to trust you and drop her inhibitions), it's incredibly easy to do. All you do is sit there, look into her eyes, nod a lot…and go back to thinking about football. I've often snuggled up to a boyfriend, thinking "What a fantastic night! Why, he's just wonderful! Funny. Articulate. Interesting. I'm hanging onto this one." Then I wake up the next day and realize it wasn't him at all, it was me! All he did was sit there and nod and I basically entertained myself with (what I thought was) a witty monologue for four hours (doubts of just how witty it really was start to surface at this point). The thing is, though, sometimes she simply won't realize it's just her who's been talking, so you can usually get away with it. On the other hand, there may just be times when you enjoy hearing what she has to say. Let's hope so.

ADORE ALL OF HER

I swear if you get these first two right, she'll be peeling grapes for you within a week. Fact: most women aren't happy with their bodies. Not even Madonna or Elle "the body" MacPherson (yes, really). The better you make her feel about her body, the better she'll be in bed (you can turn the light on for a start). Telling her over and over her butt doesn't look big won't work, but admiring less obvious sexy parts of her body will. Choose a part of her body that you really like and tell her about it. Think outside the square – how about the small of her back, inside her knee, or the curve of her hip when she's lying on her side. Just stroke your finger there and say something like "I love that part." Ignore the "Eww! That's where all the fat is" stuff. She's secretly pleased. Past lovers have told her she's got great legs, you're the first to compliment her dimples.

GET OVER THE LESBIAN THING

Every girl knows men have a thing about watching two women make love. It's harmless and sort of amusing. What's not amusing is you constantly asking us to do it. Let me reassure you: even if we're just the teensy-weensiest bit bi-curious, we'll let you know about it. OK? So no need to keep asking. If we suddenly decide we're desperate to rip the miniskirt off the office secretary, we'll let you know – afterward. (Sorry – couldn't resist.) Possibly even more annoying is the "Lesbians just need good sex with a man" argument. I can't decide which is more offensive to lesbians: the myth that "a good man" could "cure" them or the lineup of men with tongues on the floor, begging to watch them make love to their own girlfriend. While I'm sure there are some women who flee into the arms of the same sex to escape some bastard who's put their heart through a blender, most lesbians aren't there because all the men they've slept with have been duds. They're gay because they're consistently drawn both sexually and emotionally to the same sex and rarely, if ever, to the opposite sex. One night with Stud Boy isn't going to convert her.

GET FEEDBACK

Touch her half as hard as you like to be touched yourself and at half the speed: as I said, that's the general rule agreed on by most sexperts. The thing is though, we're not the ones in bed with you. It's what she likes that counts. Get feedback by suggesting you play the ratings game. She calls out a number from one to 10 (one = boring; 10 = sublime) to score how much pleasure she gets from a touch/stroke/lick on a particular part. Obviously, your challenge is to alter the touch/speed/pressure until you're close to a 10 (or she admits it's an area that just doesn't do it for her).

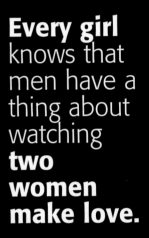

Every girl knows that men have a thing about watching **two women make love.**

SMELL NICE

I can see you rolling your eyes at this one. I know, it sounds trite, but I swear, all it takes is one smelly session and it can put you off the next six. I don't mean oversanitize yourself so you drown the naturally nice and distinctive scent of your body. Just make sure you don't reek of cigarettes and garlic, all covered up with (the ultimate turn-off) bad aftershave. I don't know if there's a scientific basis for women having a more acutely developed sense of smell but, when it comes to sniffing out week-old slices of pizza shoved under the couch, we're experts. I do know that smell is a huge part of our attraction to someone on a purely primitive level. Stuff like fresh breath matters maybe even more to us. Regarding aftershave: the trick here is to apply a small amount, so there's a hint of scent. Too much of it isn't just off-putting, it's overpowering. It makes us sneeze and it makes our eyes water. Which in turn makes our eye makeup run, so we feel less attractive and, when we feel unattractive, we definitely don't feel like sex. That definitely wasn't the result you were hoping for, now was it?

> Because it's **harder for women** to orgasm, we tend to rush to the finish line once we're on the home stretch, in case something happens to **rob us of our moment.**

EXTEND HER ORGASM POTENTIAL

Surprise, surprise! They're not all the same. Educate yourself:

Clitoral orgasms The most common type of orgasm, they result from directly stimulating the clitoris and surrounding tissue. Many sex therapists argue vehemently that all orgasms are generated via the clitoris. If she achieves orgasm through penetration only, it's because the thrusts of the penis are pulling the labia, which in turn stimulate the clitoris. Another theory is that women who orgasm with penetration only tend to have larger clitorises that are positioned high in the vagina, so are more easily stimulated in this way.

G-spot orgasms The experts pretty much agree that women who orgasm vaginally are experiencing stimulation of the anterior (front) vaginal wall, home of the infamous G-spot and A-spot and let's just accept the whole of the front vaginal wall is supersensitive, rather than argue over letters, shall we? (I'll call it G-spot though, just because it's easier and shorter than "anterior vaginal wall".) If your fantasy is to have her ejaculate, here's how. The majority of women who expel fluid do so during G-spot orgasms. Up her chances during missionary position sex by getting her to tilt her pelvis upwards, so her vulva presses flat against your pelvic bone. Pop two pillows under her butt to angle the pelvis even further.

Blended orgasms A combination of clitoral and G-spot orgasms, these are usually achieved by stimulating her clitoris with your hand during penetration particularly angled toward the front vaginal wall (see pp.112–15 for positions).

Active orgasms Just before orgasm, get her to bear down during intercourse, pushing the same muscles she'd use if she were trying to push you out of her vagina. The laws of physics then work their magic and what actually happens is the opposite: it pushes down on the penis, which squeezes it up. The result: a longer, deeper G-spot orgasm.

When you do finally **let her go all the way**, massage her lower abdomen with your hand. This stimulates **her inner clitoris** as well.

Multiple orgasms It seems that the trick to her having multiples is to keep stimulation varied and not to overstimulate any one area. The minute she's orgasmed from clitoral stimulation, remove your penis/tongue/fingers and immediately begin to stimulate her breasts, neck, lips, etc. This will keep her highly stimulated but not uncomfortably so. The latter may be the case if you continue to stimulate her clitoris.

Sequential orgasms These are what lots of people think of as multiple orgasms – more than one orgasm in one session of sex. In fact a true multiple orgasm continues in one long orgasmic wave of pleasure. The easiest way to experience one, again, is to switch stimulation lots: move from oral sex to intercourse and then back again to oral. Try stimulating different parts of her body so that she doesn't know where the next sensation is going to come from. Get her to give you lots of feedback on how it's all feeling, either verbally or through body language, to determine how fast you take it, which areas she most likes stimulated, and how quickly you move between them.

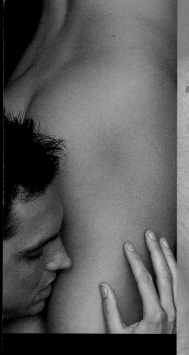

It takes the average woman around **20 minutes of oral sex** to climax, so make sure you **choose a comfortable position**.

KEEP HER HOVERING

Because it's harder for women to orgasm, we tend to rush to the finish line once we're on the home stretch, in case something happens to rob us of our moment. Next time, don't let her. The longer she hovers at the brink of orgasm, the better the resulting orgasm will be. Orgasm is simply the release of tension and blood-flow in the genitals, so make sure it's allowed to build to its peak pressure before letting go. Increase the intensity further by getting her to clench her bottom and inner thighs: it helps boost blood flow to the entire pelvic area. Let her savor the almost-but-not-quite stage by switching between intense and direct stimulation (like oral sex) and milder, nongenital stimulation (kissing or touching her breasts). When you do finally let her go all the way, massage her lower abdomen with your hand. This stimulates her inner clitoris as well. The part you see is merely the tip – the clitoris is actually around 9 inches (23cm) of highly sensitive erectile tissue, extending along the front side of the vaginal wall.

WORK OUT WITH HER

Except I'm not talking weights or jogging: this is a gym workout for your genitals. They're officially called "kegel" exercises and they work on toning up your "sex" or "love" muscle: the PC or pubococcygeous (hers) or bulbocavernosus (yours). These muscles control the walls of the vagina and penis respectively. Basically, the more toned they are and the greater control you have over them, the better sex will be. They're also remarkably effective at helping her turn herself on. When women contract their kegel or PC muscles, they cause the walls of the vagina to contract, which in turn causes the walls to excrete fluid and lubricate in readiness for sex. The clitoris rests on these muscles, so stronger PC muscles often lead to stronger sensations during orgasm. The same thing happens when you do kegels: you'll begin to experience an erection. It's called self-excitation and it's incredibly useful for impotence, incompatible sex drives, and general who-can-be-bothered-screwing blues. There are lots of variations of genital workouts but this one's by far the best. Go on, get squeezing!

- To identify the muscle: the next time you urinate, allow a small amount of urine to pass, then cut off the flow. The muscle you're using is your "sex" muscle. This is the muscle we're aiming to develop ultimate control of. She'll feel a tightening inside the vagina. You'll feel it behind your testicles, just in front of your anus.
- Squeeze and hold this muscle as often as you can. She should picture bringing the walls of the vagina together; you visualize pulling your testicles together or pulling upward on your penis. Try to work up to sets

of 10, then 25. Try to hold and squeeze the muscle for several seconds at a time. OK, that's the easy part. Yes, really.

● Now we need to gain control of them during intercourse. For her: she should insert a thin cylindrical object (like a minitampon or her finger) and pull on the muscle as she did before. She needs to keep practicing until she feels her muscles gripping it tightly, then insert a larger object (or two fingers) and continue. The idea is to keep increasing the size of the object until it's around the same size as your penis. For him: keep flexing and holding until you can move your penis back and forth toward and away from your body. Masters of the technique will be able to move it from side to side as well. As for women, it's a lot harder to control this muscle during penetration, but practice makes perfect!

GIVE GREAT ORAL

Tips on how much women love oral sex, and how to do it right, are scattered throughout the book (like on every page). Just in case you haven't gotten the hint (or have flicked straight to this part), let me repeat myself: the surest way to give her an orgasm is through (good) oral sex. Lots of women only orgasm through oral sex. By the way, it takes the average woman around 20 minutes of oral sex to climax, so make sure you choose a comfortable position.

EXPERIMENT TOGETHER

The perception is that women aren't as interested in sexual experimentation as men. Initially, in new relationships, it's probably true. If she likes you, she's not going to pull out the red leather corset and whip just yet, in case you freak out and run away. Once she realizes you won't judge her and she trusts you, don't be surprised if she's as eager to conquer unexplored territories as you are. Take anal sex. True, many women blanch at the thought, but plenty don't. Here's how to proceed if she's willing: gently stroke the outside of her anus, checking her response and ensuring that she's comfortable before inserting a well-lubricated finger. Work up to two fingers over a few sessions and she'll have a pretty good idea whether she wants to take things further. I warn you though, don't kid yourself or her: it will hurt the first time. Use tons of lubricant and take it very, very slowly before working up to full penetration. At no point continue if it hurts too much. Something else to think about: anal sex is the highest risk activity for transmission of STDs (sexually transmitted diseases). The trauma and stretching of penetration can lead to tears and cuts in the fragile wall of the rectum, which make everything alarmingly vulnerable to infection. You may not want to use a condom when having vaginal sex, but it's putting both the health of you and your partner at risk to attempt anal sex without one. Don't even think of touching her vagina before you change condoms (or discard altogether); the risk of infection is just too high. Condoms designed for vaginal sex are much thinner, so ensure that you're using one of the extrastrong variety, manufactured to resist the strains of anal sex. If you'd like to get tested for any STD , visit your local doctor or ask for a referral to your nearest STD clinic. Or if you're too shy, call any major hospital and ask if they have an STD clinic with a walk-in service. When you're getting tested, ask them to take anal swabs and explain that you have had anal sex. Yes, I know, embarrassing, but believe me, they've heard it all before.

Sure-thing sex positions

Up your chances for an orgasm every time

If you're one of those lucky women who are able to orgasm purely from intercourse then I'm very pleased for you. You can now go back to whatever else it was you were doing (like moving your house a few feet to the left). Anyway, enough about you already. This is for the rest of us: the 90-odd percent of women who have the majority of our orgasm quota through oral sex or masturbation.

Not that we're complaining or jealous, mind you. OK, we are. Because as much as orgasms are delicious any way you can get them, it would be pretty nice to have one during intercourse, when he's having one, too.

The point of all these sexual positions is to up your orgasm quota by using a combination of techniques to hit both internal and external hot spots. Never one to leave much to chance, I suggest we hedge our bets by mounting this campaign on two fronts: with words and action. Like, how about we debunk the myth and let him in on the secret, eh? You know, the one about the penis being the almighty satisfier. Because it's…well, just not true. Be honest. If you can only climax during intercourse when he's stroking your clitoris as well, tell him! Explain that it's not his fault but that lots of women are built that way and that it's a matter of biology, and has nothing to do with his sexual technique. If he's got a problem, tell him to take it up with God, failing that, Mother Nature. Once he's recovered, give him a biology lesson.

Does he know exactly where your clitoris is? Has he had a good look at it in broad daylight? Don't get all shy on me puhleeze! It's dark down there and it's easy to lose his bearings during different intercourse positions. I'm not saying that you lie down spread-eagle on the kitchen table just as the next-door neighbor stops by for morning coffee, but it is a very good idea to have the lights on at some point when he's giving you oral sex. Get him onside and clued up, then you can move on to trying your luck with these little gems. Now, I freely admit that one or two of these positions aren't just advanced but damn near impossible – unless you've got the flexibility of an acrobat and body confidence of a supermodel. But never mind: you can always pretend that this is what you get up to when drunk at a dinner party! By the way, I've geared this section to women, simply because it's easier to address one of you at a time when you're talking about legs facing this way and arms the other!

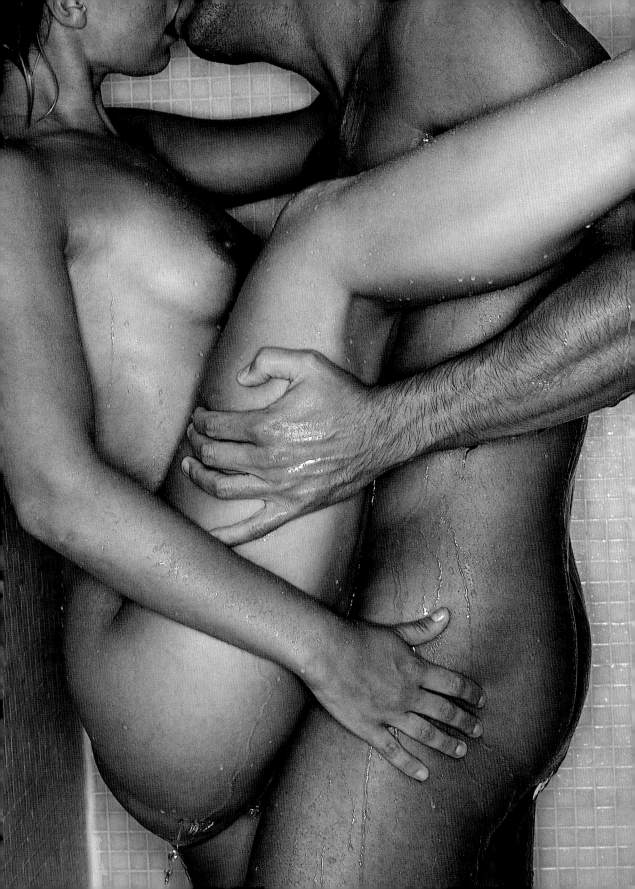

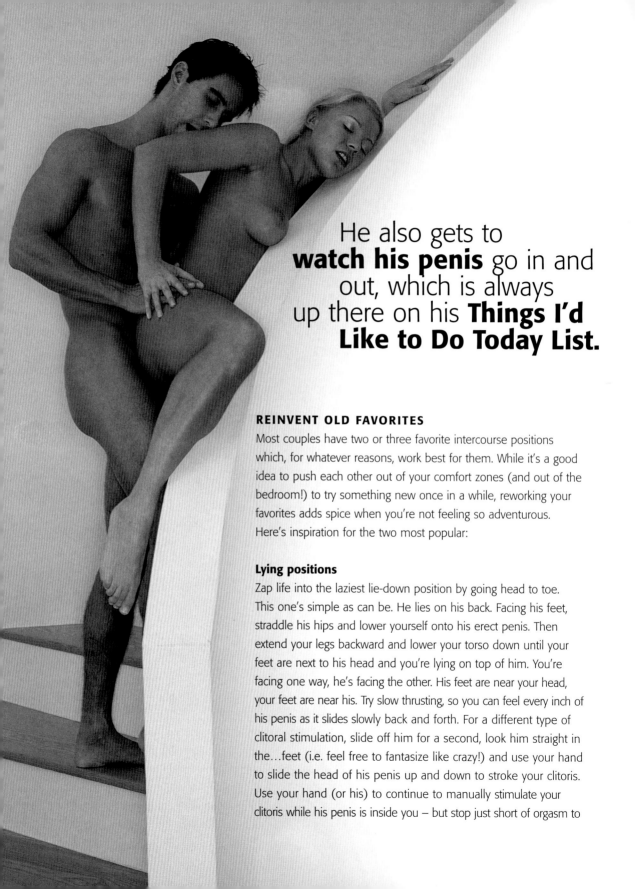

He also gets to **watch his penis** go in and out, which is always up there on his **Things I'd Like to Do Today List.**

REINVENT OLD FAVORITES

Most couples have two or three favorite intercourse positions which, for whatever reasons, work best for them. While it's a good idea to push each other out of your comfort zones (and out of the bedroom!) to try something new once in a while, reworking your favorites adds spice when you're not feeling so adventurous. Here's inspiration for the two most popular:

Lying positions

Zap life into the laziest lie-down position by going head to toe. This one's simple as can be. He lies on his back. Facing his feet, straddle his hips and lower yourself onto his erect penis. Then extend your legs backward and lower your torso down until your feet are next to his head and you're lying on top of him. You're facing one way, he's facing the other. His feet are near your head, your feet are near his. Try slow thrusting, so you can feel every inch of his penis as it slides slowly back and forth. For a different type of clitoral stimulation, slide off him for a second, look him straight in the…feet (i.e. feel free to fantasize like crazy!) and use your hand to slide the head of his penis up and down to stroke your clitoris. Use your hand (or his) to continue to manually stimulate your clitoris while his penis is inside you – but stop just short of orgasm to let his thrusting trigger off the orgasm itself – and you've done what's officially called the "bridge maneuver." What this does is form a "bridge" between clitoral stimulation (how most women orgasm) and a penetrative orgasm (how most men would like them to). Smart girl!

Girls on top

Ask him to sit up on the bed, his legs extended straight out in front of him. Climb on top, cowgirl style, and let him penetrate. Now fall back as far as you can until the top of your head is just resting on the bed. Reach backward with your hands until you can grasp his feet. Not only does your stomach look amazingly thin in this position, it's also easy to turn it into a killer workout if it suddenly reminds you that you should be at the gym, rather than lying around having sex. Instead of straddling him and resting on your knees, squat instead so your feet are on the bed. Stay leaning forward, then you do all the work – as in thrusting – and the only way to do this is to lift your heels and use those thigh muscles. Whatever, this position is bouncy, sexy sex – perfect for teasing him. Switch from fast up-and-down action before shifting gears and going for wide, circular motions. Will he like it? Excuse me? Your body is on full display so he gets to admire a full-frontal view because this position lays it all right out in front of him! He also gets to watch his penis go in and out, which is always up there on his Things I'd Like to Do Today List. (And one reason why this position is not such a great idea for Johnny-come-quickly's, because they'll lose it within seconds.)

Turn your back on him

The front wall of the vagina is incredibly sensitive – which is why rear-entry feels great for women. Here's three good reasons to sacrifice the benefits of face-to-face positions (like kissing) for other delights (orgasms). Thought I might convince you!

- **To activate a G-spot orgasm** Him-from-behind positions alter the angle of the vagina and give him a direct shot. Positions like The Swivel (see p.113) are ideal. Try it by arching your back as far as you can, and widening your legs so his penis has perfect access. If he's hitting the right spot and continues to thrust, the first reaction you may have is that you feel you need to pee because the G-spot is near the urethra (through which urine passes). Hang on (in all senses) and the sensation will pass and turn into an orgasmic wave that washes over you.

- **To get a good feel** Him-behind positions leave your hands free to stimulate his testicles and perineum (the smooth area between his testicles and anus). Meanwhile, he can stroke your back, bottom, and lower stomach. You get to set the pace and rhythm, to regulate the depth of penetration and to generally be the dominant one. It's also a great position to give yourself a helping hand at crucial points because it's easy to reach down and stimulate your clitoris.

- **For fantasy paradise** There's no eye contact so both of you are free to fantasize about anyone and anything you like (without feeling guilty when opening one eye to see your partner gazing lovingly into yours). The rear-entry position is wonderfully primitive, so perfect for those slightly wild, don't-even-admit-to-your-best-friend-type-of fantasies that suit "dirty" sex.

SIT-DOWN SEX

How to do it

He lies on his back and gets into the old "bicycle" exercise position (resting on his shoulders, his hips and butt in the air, weight resting on his elbows, and hands holding hips high). You stand and face away from him and lower yourself onto his penis by sitting down on his butt. His feet then rest against your back, while you rest your fingers on the back of his thighs for balance.

Why you'll love it

Yes, this one is a little tricky! His penis needs to be bent back and through his legs, which is why a semierection works best. Why attempt it? He might not love it but you will. You're in the driver's seat (literally) so can custom-order your orgasm by controlling the depth of penetration and speed of thrusting.

THE HOOK

How to do it

You're lying on your back, he's on top. Hook your legs up over his shoulders for deeper penetration and to give him complete control.

Why you'll love it

If he's not terribly well-endowed, it's a good position for maximum deep penetration.

A tip to remember for this and other positions: crossing your ankles (in this case behind his neck) helps tighten the vaginal canal. It's also a great way to squeeze him in and make him feel fuller inside you. The scrotum brushes against your buttocks with each stroke. You can reach forward to stroke or cup his testicles, while he can do wonderful things to your breasts with his hands. The blood will have rushed to extremities like your nipples, which makes them highly sensitive.

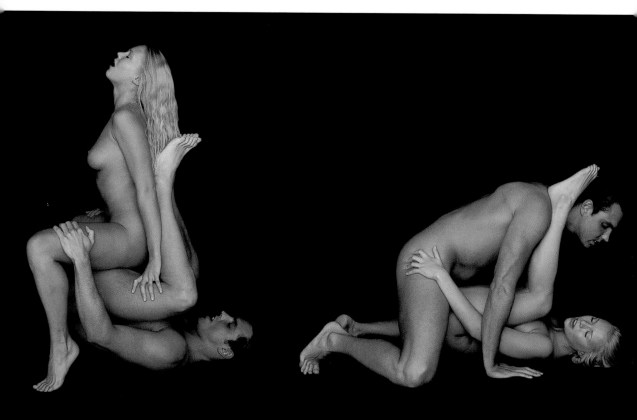

THE SLIDE

How to do it

He kneels on a hard surface, keeping his back straight, in a praying position. You lie in front of him, genitals facing him. He then lifts your legs up to his shoulders, so your weight is supported on your shoulders. Holding his erection downward, he then penetrates you. He holds you in position by wrapping his arms around your upper thighs.

Why you'll love it

This works because it's a position where he penetrates shallowly. And – gosh! how terribly tactful is Mother Nature! – all the vaginal nerve endings are located within an inch or so of the vaginal entrance. The reason why this position works: he's focusing on your supersensitive nerve endings with what also happens to be his most sensitive part – the head of his penis.

THE SWIVEL

How to do it

You're on top, then through a series of moves, you turn around while he's still inside you and end up facing the opposite way. So start by riding him, rodeo-style. Then, using your hands to steady yourself, lift one leg over your body and begin to turn sideways. Continue rotating, stopping at intervals for a few thrusts, until you're facing away from him.

Why you'll love it

He gets a unique "corkscrew" feeling on his penis while you turn around, and is simultaneously treated to a revolving-restaurant-type view of your body. His erection points out instead of up, which is an instant arousal upper. You can vary the thrusting to make things even more interesting. Grind into him slowly, then suddenly speed up, or vary the depth of penetration.

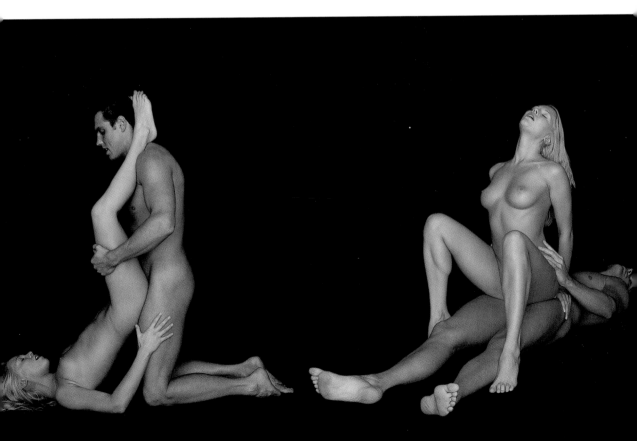

UPSIDE-DOWN SEX

How to do it

Both stand facing each other. You jump up and wrap your legs around his waist and arms around his neck. Let him penetrate, then very slowly and carefully let go and let your body fall backward until you're in a handstand position with your palms on the floor, facing away from him. He supports you by holding your waist and buttocks. Yes, you do need to be flexible but it's actually not as difficult as it sounds (and you've got to admit, it looks damn impressive!).

Why you'll love it

It's called inversion: him taking you head down. Because the blood literally rushes to your head, it builds pressure in the veins of the face and neck, producing startling sensations on orgasm. Oh, and it's great for your balance and gives your abs a workout. Beats the gym!

THE INTERLOCK

How to do it

Start by getting into the missionary position. He then sits up and brings both legs forward, one at a time, so the soles of his feet are flat on the bed. His knees are bent and he's facing you. He then leans back and supports himself on his hands. You sit up and support yourself on your hands. Put your ankles on his shoulders and lift your hips as high as possible.

Why you'll love it

This position's good for aiming at the A-spot (the Anterior Fornex Erogenous). This hot spot was accidentally discovered in 1996 by scientists trying to find a cure for vaginal dryness. They were astonished to find 95 percent of women became massively turned on when this area was stimulated. It's a smooth, extremely sensitive spot halfway between your G-spot and your cervix.

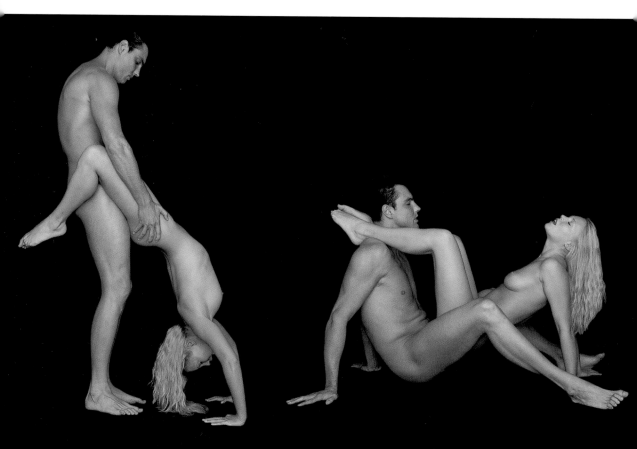

THE WALL THRUST

How to do it

You lean with your back against a wall; he stands in front of you. Now jump up and wrap your legs around his waist and put your arms around his neck, keeping your back and head against the wall for stability. He penetrates in this position, legs apart, hands holding on to your thighs and bottom.

Why you'll love it

Because he's holding you, he feels a real sense of power and potency. He can also maintain an erection for longer when standing up because the blood is needed elsewhere in his body, so his erection isn't as intense. This isn't bad news. It means he's in control enough to spend time concentrating on your pleasure and the slow teasing and buildup makes his orgasm positively explosive when it actually happens.

THE STARFISH

How to do it

You both lie on the bed, heads in opposite directions. Scissor your legs so he can penetrate, then hang on to each other's hands for leverage.

Why you'll love it

This technique is perfect to achieve a grinding pressure movement, advocated by the CAT (Coital Alignment Technique). Given that the in-out, in-out motion of thrusting during intercourse does little to keep the pressure constant on the clitoris – which is what's needed for orgasm – the CAT technique works on the principle that instead of moving apart, you should push your hips together and maintain pressure on the clitoris as you rock back and forth. (Purrrr!). Arch your backs and move away from each other to allow deeper penetration or adjust the angle so he's hitting the right spots.

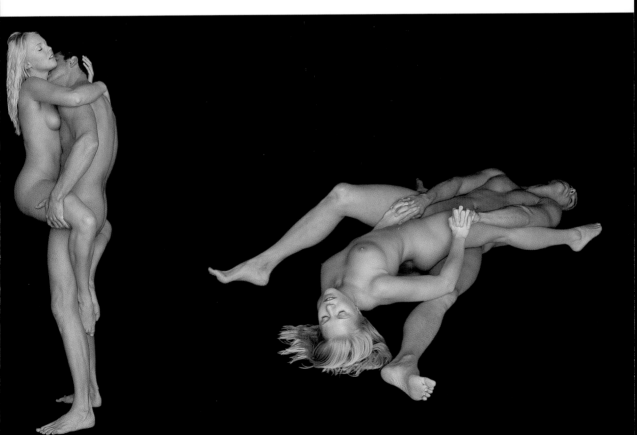

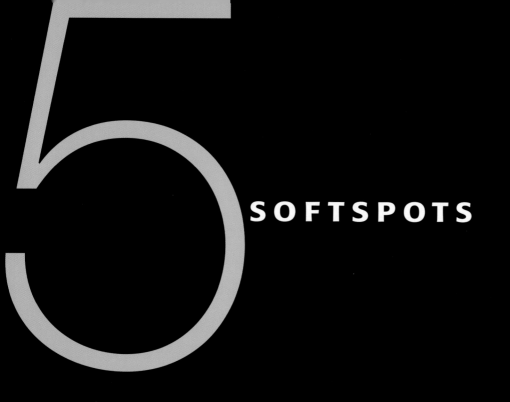

5

SOFTSPOTS

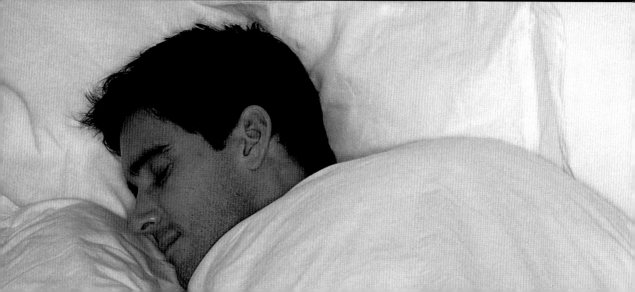

What to do when your parts **don't fit**, answers to the world's most **humiliating sex** questions, a five-part guide for superforeplay – and (gulp!) lessons on how to tell a lover they're **bad in bed**.

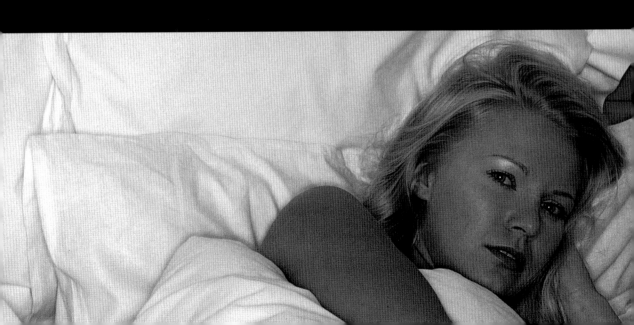

Be a better bonk
The five-part guide to superforeplay

Don't believe the headline (a cunning ploy to lure the all-roads-lead-to-intercourse-people), this is about everything BUT the lay. Want to have mind-blowing sex? It can't be done without memorable foreplay. No, really. The right foreplay can put the pash back into passion and turn your mattress into molten lava (oh come on, what more do I have to promise to win you over?). Now whether that involves dribbling cream all over her *derrière* (and wouldn't you kill for the one opposite?), or playing policewoman with the handcuffs, is up to you. What this should help to do is whet your appetites, stimulate the senses, and give those stalled imaginations a jump start. If you're really eager to up the intimacy level, take turns as suggested, and work through all of the following exercises over a six-week period.

TOUCH
For her
- Generally, it's a good idea to start with the nonsensitive parts and work up to the most sensitive. The genitals and other obvious hot spots get attention last, not first.
- Ask yourself "Where and how can I touch her in a way/place she's never been touched before?"
- When you're next hugging, pull away from her and stand back a little so you can see her whole body. Then touch it slowly and reverently, like it's the very first time and it's something you never, ever dreamed would be possible. Keep her at arm's length and let your eyes alternate between intense, direct eye contact and gazing at the body part you're touching. The whole effect is of you marveling at her body.

For both of you
- Let different body parts take center stage by focusing your attention on different parts during different sessions. Session 1. breasts/chest get top billing; 2. neck and arms; 3. back and shoulders; 4. thighs – inside and back of; 5. tummy and lower abdomen; 6. the genitals finally get a turn.

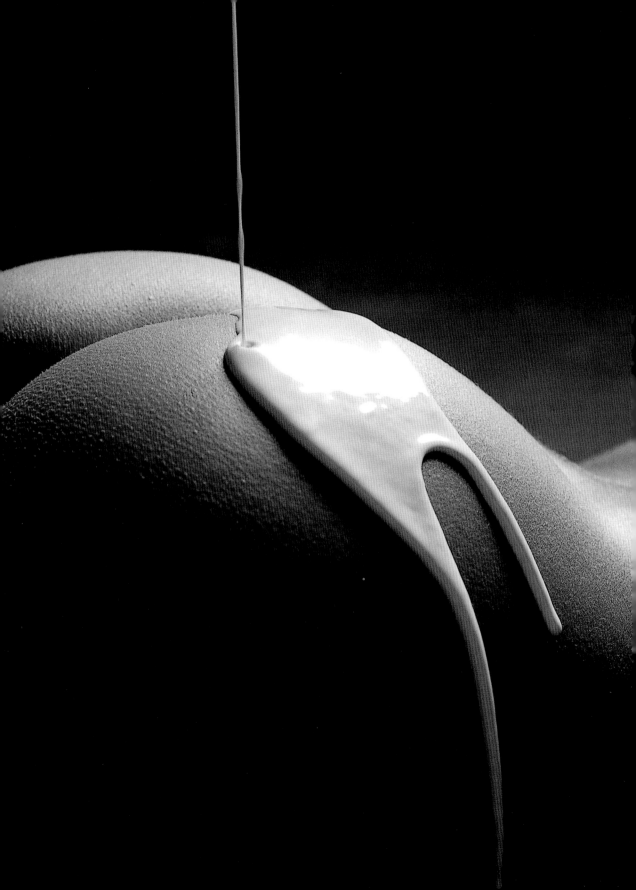

TORMENT
For him

- Take him lingerie shopping. Hold his hand and make him cruise around the underwear department of all the major stores, drag him into speciality shops like Victoria's Secret or Frederick's of Hollywood. Then take him home, remove all your clothes, take the shirt off his back, and put it on yours, held together by one button only. Proceed to cook dinner, bending over lots, while he chats to you in the kitchen. (Bet you burn it all.)
- Hold his erection firmly in one hand while you use your other to stroke his chest and stomach, gradually getting closer to his genitals. Maintain eye contact the whole time and watch him squirm.
- Make a rule of keeping your clothes on for as long as possible. When you do remove them, do it piece by piece, not all at once. Slow everything up. Extend the torture by wearing sheer underwear: he can see the good parts through the fabric but there's still a barrier between him and your flesh.

For both of you

- Each choose some erotic reading material then perch at either end of the couch facing each other with only your calves entwined. Now read the good bits outloud to each other, maintaining eye contact but not touching with your hands.

EXPLORE
For her

- Stop seeing sex as a series of steps toward an end goal (intercourse/orgasm). Stay focused on the here and now, and not where you're going. Happiness is in the journey and all that. Simple advice but it'll make an extraordinary difference to her satisfaction levels.
- Vary the way she has orgasms by breaking out of the comfort zone. Most of us orgasm in the way that's easiest and ignore alternatives. She only orgasms through oral sex? Ban it for a month! Yes, she'll hate you. But not if you master other techniques. Her body will resist initially, but then respond with: "I'm not getting any tongue action here, I might as well try to get used to his fingers instead." By varying her means to orgasm, you up the chances of her becoming multiorgasmic.

For both of you

- Have sense-ational sex: dull one sense each time you have sex to heighten the others. Here's your deprivation device schedule: Sight session: blindfolds. Hearing session: earplugs. Touch session: each of you have your hands tied behind your back (it's awkward tying theirs when yours are tied already, but it can be done!). Taste session: no mouth contact at all. Smell session:

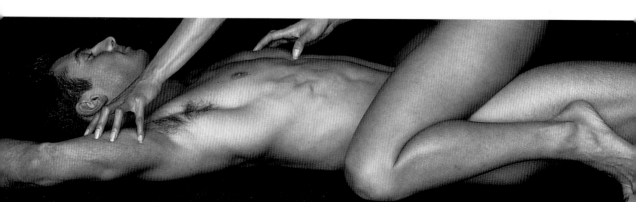

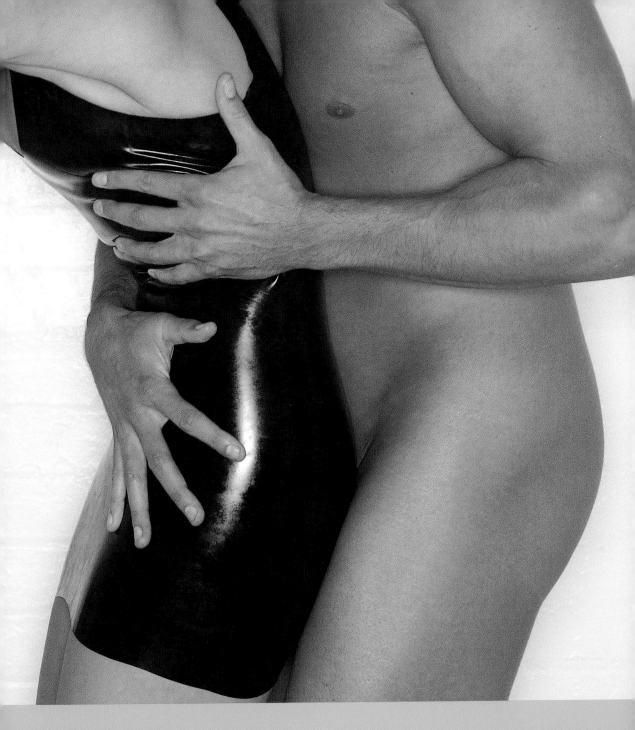

Extend the torture by wearing sheer underwear: he can see the good bits **through the fabric** but there's still a barrier between **him and your flesh**.

ummmm…OK, I admit defeat (I draw the line at holding each others' noses). Instead, do the opposite for this one and focus on smell (burn some aromatherapy oils or massage each other with scented lotions).

EXCITE

For her

- Do it anywhere but the bedroom to instantly up the frisk factor. Lure him into the bathroom to watch you shave your legs – then let him shave the rest of you.
- Have phone sex during his lunch hour. Wait until the rest of your office nips out for a sandwich, then close your door and call him with creative carnal confessions (make them up or pick up a dirty magazine on the way to work that morning).
- Invite him in for a sexy food experience. The phallic-shaped ones (cucumbers, carrots), you eat suggestively in front of him. The spreadable variety (chocolate mousse, cream, honey) are dipped and smeared over his nipples, penis, and testicles. Try licking them off by running your tongue in figure eights around his testicles.

For both of you

- Link sex and smell. According to research, memories of sex are the quickest to fade because the feelings come from a primitive part of the brain that has little capacity to store memory. Smell, on the other hand, has a powerful effect on memory. Wear a particular perfume each time you have sex or burn an aromatherapy oil and your sex memories will be much easier to recall. The next time you smell the scent, your brain instantly conjures up how fabulous it felt – encouraging you to go for a repeat, even if you are both dog tired.

PLAY

For her

- One way to concentrate on her naked is to draw an erotic picture of her. Remember the scene in *Titanic* when Leonardo draws Kate, as she reclines, naked except for THE necklace, in the cabin she shares with her fiancée? (Naughty Kate!) This works on two levels: you get to feast your eyes on her body and really see it; she feels admired and beautiful. It doesn't really matter whether the end product looks like it's been painted by Picasso on acid (but if it does, call the MOMA), it's the process we're interested in.
- Jump on her just as you're both about to rush out the door, late for dinner/a party/your mom's for Sunday dinner. Pause, with your hand on the doorknob, let your eyes travel over her body and say "Hang on a minute." Then look at her and say "Does it matter if we're three minutes late?" Putting a time limit on things ups the tension and makes everything urgent. In all the right ways.

For both of you

- Break the routine. Do the opposite of what you did the last time you had sex. It was in the morning? Then do it at night. In the bedroom? Try the kitchen. You did it missionary position? Tonight it's rear entry.

Toy with each other

Remember the toy box you had as a kid? Here's
what to put in your very adult version:

- **Essentials** Personal lubricant, condoms.
- **Gadgets** A vibrator, handcuffs, serious sex aids,
  a Polaroid camera, erotic videos.
- **Get-ups** Dress-up clothes for acting out fantasies.
- **Giggles** Edible goodies (anything that can be
  licked, sucked, or rubbed off), sexy board games,
  silly sex toys.
- **Good reads** Sexy books and magazines.
- **Romance revivers** Candles, aromatherapy, and
  massage oils.
- **Tie-ups** Silk stockings and scarves, blindfolds.

She only **orgasms through oral sex**?
Ban it for a month. Yes, **she'll hate you**.
But she won't later, when she's **multiorgasmic**.

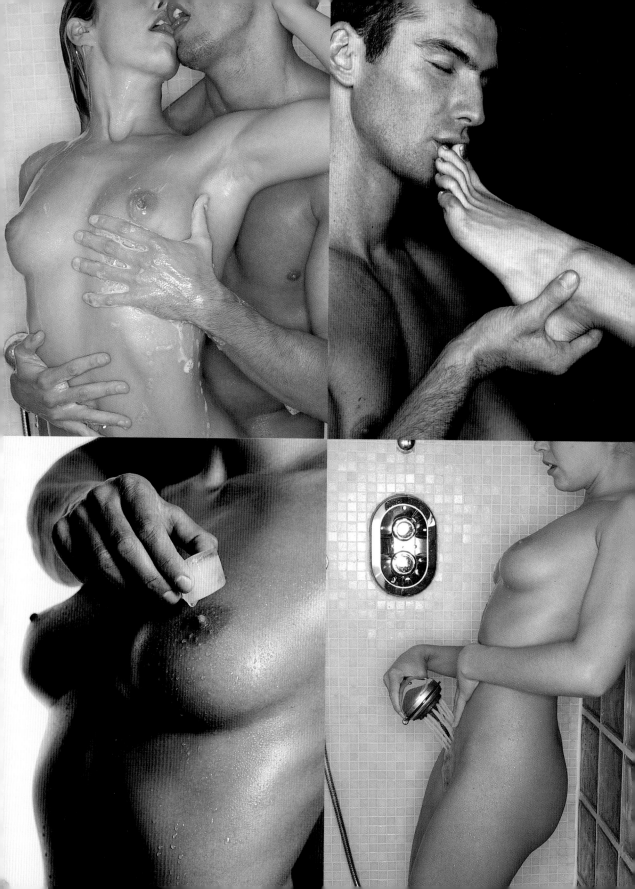

The passion plan

What, when, and how much foreplay you need depends on how long you've been together. On that very first night, a look can turn you to jelly; six years later, it takes a little more to make you melt. Being fabulous at foreplay hinges a lot on doing the unexpected so that sex feels spontaneous, but anticipation and creative planning can be just as sexy.

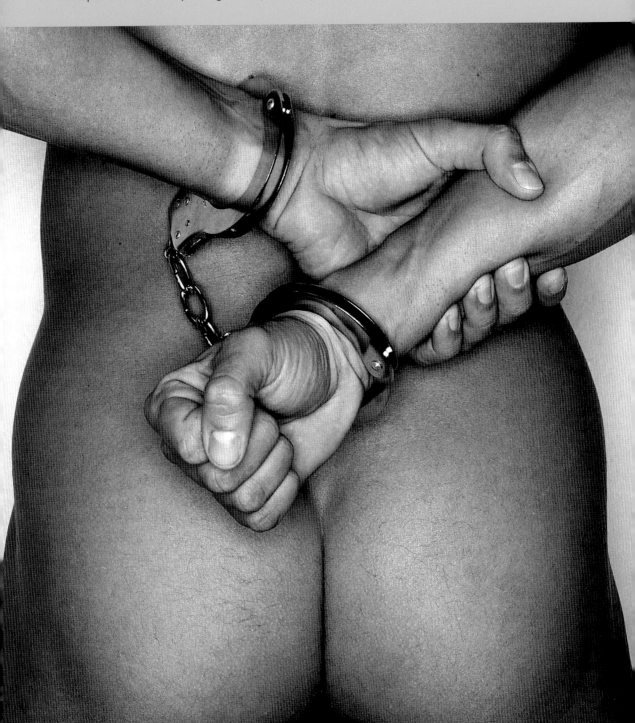

"Honey, we need to talk"

...and it's not about washing the dishes

Look, I'm with you: telling someone you love that having sex with them sucks certainly isn't the easiest thing in the world to do. But, if you do it, I can guarantee you two things instantly. No 1: It's not as bad as you think; No 2: It will make such a difference to your sex life, you will immediately pledge your firstborn child, life savings (maybe the snazzy red sports car you've got tucked away in the garage?) to the person responsible for making you do it. Which would be me. (All right then, I'll take the car.) Seriously! Crack the code on this one and you're set for a lifetime of great loving.

Even better news: it really isn't that difficult if you follow one simple rule. The secret to telling someone they're the worst lover you've ever had is...not to. Focus on what you want, not what you don't, and you'll find the solution without ever owning up to having a problem! Confused? Keep reading and I promise it will all make sense.

THE OUT-OF-BED ACTION PLAN

Figure out what you want Start by focusing on yourself, not your partner. Make a list of 10 things you want more of in bed, 10 things you want less of, and 10 new things you'd like to try. Finding it harder than you think? This is the mistake lots of people make. Saying "I hate it when you do that" isn't much help unless you suggest something you'd like them to do instead. You have to know what you want in bed in order to get it. One final check before you proceed further: how specific are your lists? Do they simply and clearly spell out exactly what you want, and for how long? Your partner is not a mind reader. Loving you does not mean they know exactly what you need to turn you on at that exact moment. Let me repeat that: your partner is NOT a mind reader. Which is why it's a good idea to...

Let him in on the secret There's little point in only you knowing how to give you pleasure, is there? Here's where you open your mouth and – shock, horror! – tell your partner about it!! Choose a time when you're both getting along reasonably well (call me an alcoholic but I always think a good time is when you're both a little merry and having a laugh), then simply bring the subject of sex up. "Gosh, I forgot to tell you! Remember Susan? The girl I used to go to school with?" (A complete lie – all of it.)

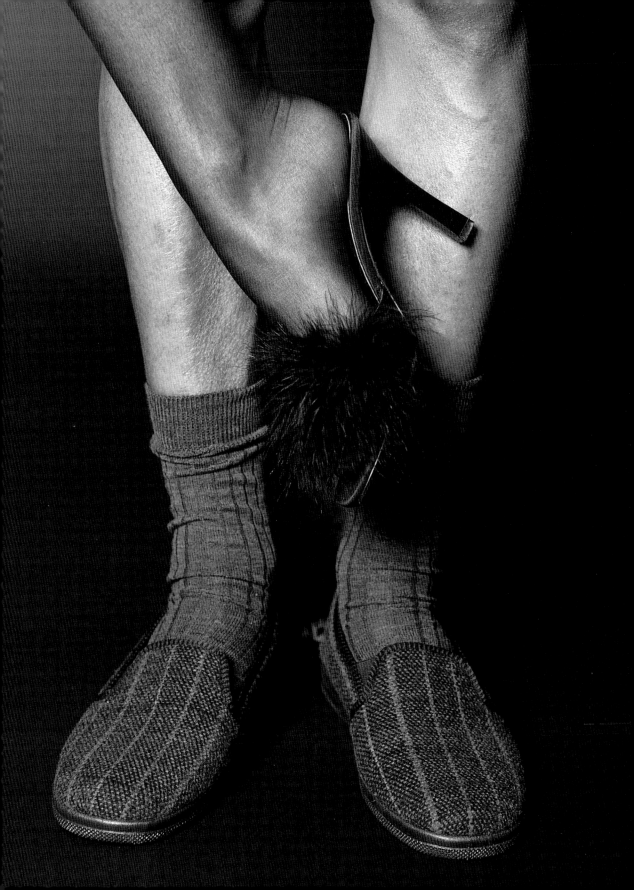

Sex life's all a big mess?
7 steps to salvation

1. **Don't fight change** Your taste in clothes varies over time; so do your sexual tastes and needs. Keep your partner up-to-date and they won't feel threatened – or left behind.

2. **Work on your self-esteem** The happier you are with who you are, the more likely you are to speak up. Check that there's no power imbalance in your relationship. The one who makes the sexual moves is usually the one who calls the shots.

3. **Build intimacy outside the bedroom** Let your partner see the '"real" you – especially the silly, awkward parts. If you feel like doing Britney impressions, dancing around the living room, do it! The more often they see the not-so-glam-or-in-control you, the more they'll relax.

4. **Remove any blame** If the problem is that one of you wants sex more, don't persecute the "less sexy" partner or accuse the other one of being a "sex maniac." It's no one's fault. It's a problem the two of you have, so solve it as a couple: together.

5. **Both figure out what you're upset about** Think long and hard on your own before coming together to talk about it. Try to think of solutions, not just the problem. If you're upset because he's not spending enough time on foreplay, spell out exactly what you'd like more of. Then talk it through.

6. **Don't avoid sex; keep on having it** Most sex problems turn into long-term dramas when the couple avoids the bedroom and refuse to admit there's a problem.

7. **Break your relationship routine** Start off small: suggest you go to the movies instead of renting a video. Have sex in the guest room instead of your own. New experiences leave us feeling refreshed and pay dividends.

"Well, I found out today that she's left her husband and run off with a younger man – purely for sex!" (I know, complete bullshit – just keep going.) "Anyway, I started thinking, I hope you won't run out on me because you aren't happy with our sex life. And then I thought, we really should put more effort into it. There are lots of new things we could try in bed and I'd hate you not to be happy…" Get the idea? You're opening up a two-way discussion about sex: both of you talking as a team instead of you pointing the finger. In fact, you're actually in the background and giving them center stage. Maybe even insinuating they'd have more to complain about than you would! Hold the indignance – it's the end result that counts.

Work from the positive This is the crucial part. Always start by telling your partner what they're doing right before moving on to what they're doing wrong. Talk about what you want more of in bed, not less. I don't care if the only thing she does right is turn the lights off. Whispering "I love the way you make it all dark and sexy" is still better than "Oh for God's sake, when is it NOT a fat day?!" Lying helps. Say, "Wow! That felt great when your tongue hit that spot – go back there!" (and give instructions). It's kinder and more constructive than saying her tongue is so far off target it was in the next room. Master the art of criticizing without wounding feelings.

BACK IN THE SACK
Put your money where your mouth is (or should now be) by reinforcing your words with body language. Continue the good work by learning to:

Use your hands If they're still not getting it right (and they're probably not yet because words can only explain so much), redirect. Use your hands to move his/her hand/mouth/hips to where you'd like them to go. It's pointless (not to mention a complete waste of time that could be spent enjoying yourself) to just lie there and hope they'll eventually hit the spot. Instead, reach down and show them where/what/how hard you want him/her to be.

Back it up with body language Praise them vocally and with your body when they get it right. Make it so obvious that even the neighbors know. Apply the same technique when they do something you DON'T like. Show zero enthusiasm so they get the message: "Honey, that feels about as pleasurable as a getting a Pap smear when they haven't warmed up the steel thing."

Avoid judging others by your own behavior If we respond to something a certain way, we assume everyone does. Wrong! We're all individuals. Take noise in bed, for example. The world divides into three types – those who scream, groan, moan, and generally wake up the neighbors from the first kiss to the last thrust (about 20 percent); those who are generally quiet but fairly vocal during the climax part, emitting grunts, sighs, and involuntary moans on orgasm (about 60 percent); and those who keep quiet no matter what (about 20 percent). Lara Croft could burst through the computer screen, fall on her knees and deliver, and he'd still stay silent. So don't take it personally if your partner does fall into the last category, OK? Why are some people vocal and others aren't? It's more to do with upbringing, past experience, and personality than enjoyment of the experience. It doesn't mean they're not enjoying it; it just means they're more quiet/embarrassed/inhibited/private about sex than you are. So even if they're not writhing on the bed screaming Yes! Yes! Yes!, it doesn't mean they're not melting on the inside.

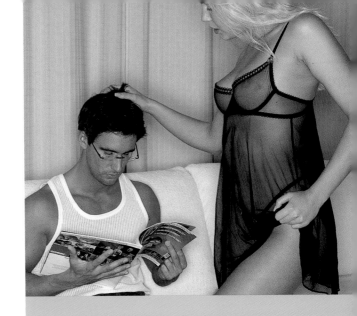

Techniques to get you talking

- **The five-minute confessional** Set an alarm clock for five minutes then put it out of sight. One person is "talker," the other "listener." Then each takes turns doing just that. The "listener" cannot interrupt until the alarm rings. Reset the alarm and they get to talk for five minutes. It's much easier to talk if you know you won't be interrupted. It's much easier to listen if you know you'll have your say soon after. Five minutes is a long time.

- **The alien game** This gives you an excuse to start from scratch because, well…one of you is from outer space. Pretend one of you is an alien and the other an earthling. The alien has never had sex before, never seen a human naked, so has no idea how to touch them or what to do. The "earthling" has to instruct the alien, very specifically, on how to arouse them. If you're the alien, start asking the million sex questions you would have buzzing around in your head: Does this feel good? Why does it feel good? Is this even better? Why? As the earthling, you explain why touching a certain part of you in a certain way makes you aroused.

Untouchables vs. insatiables
They want it; you don't – or vice versa

Hands up who had ohmigod-we've-ruined-yet-another-set-of-sheets sex last night? OK, how about reasonably good sex that left you with a rather smug post-coital glow? Hmmm. All right, how many of you fantasize more about sleeping in your bed than bouncing around on it? Well hullo and welcome to the 21st century: a time when most of us give career and kids number one billing in life – and sex bottom priority, by being the last thing we do at night.

This is how more than half the population cope sexually with stressful jobs and the dramas of everyday life: they don't, basically. Others react to the pressure by using sex as a stress-release rather than pleasure-enhancer – and end up with a different, though equally bad, set of problems: soulless sex. Then, to really help matters, these two different types of people decide to get together and hook up romantically. Now isn't that a great idea?

I've said this once and I'll keep on saying it: when you're choosing a partner, if you can possibly swing it, try really hard to choose one with the same sexual appetite as you. Because mismatched libidos – one wanting sex more or less than the other – is one of the main sex problems affecting couples today. A trillion factors dictate whether we're a high or low libido person: pressure and stress, medications, past history, possible previous sexual traumas, our partner's lovemaking skills, general health – all play a part. Genes too. Some people just don't have terribly many sexual thoughts, feelings, or fantasies. They seriously could chat to the world's most desired sex object and come away thinking, "What a jolly nice person! Gosh! Who'd have thought they also have problems with their golf swing!" while the rest of us have mentally undressed them, slammed them up against the nearest wall, had our wicked way and 25 orgasms each before "Hello!" even escaped our lips. Whichever camp you fall into is irrelevant in relationship terms: if your sex drives are unequal, then you're in for a bumpy ride, with friction and resentment around every corner. It's a problem that can ultimately ruin even the best relationships – but there is loads to be done to even up the sexual scales. For all the Tweedledums who didn't quite manage to match with their sexual Tweedledees, this is for you…

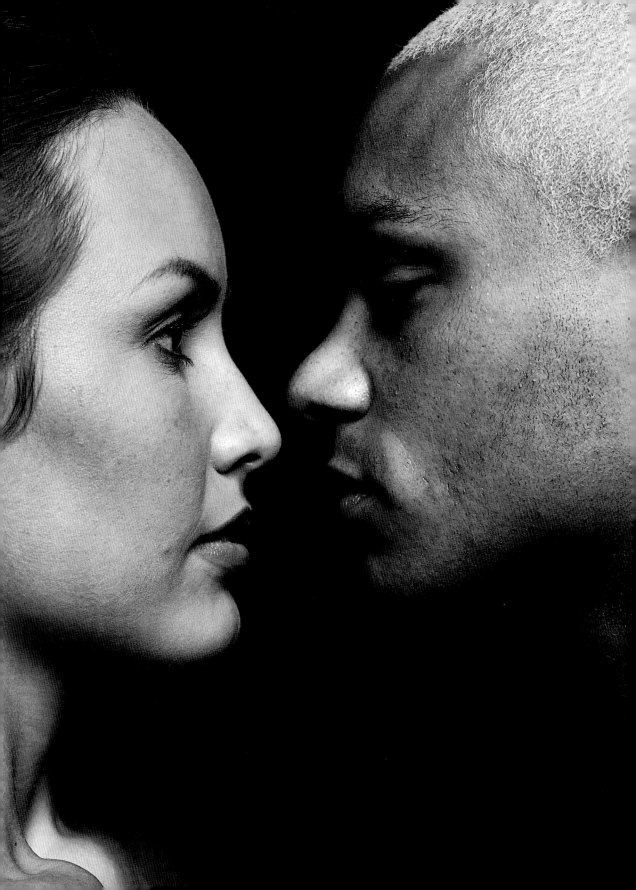

THE FIX-ITS: THEY WANT IT MORE THAN YOU DO

- **Get a good night's sleep** Impaired sleep leads to a reduction in testosterone, the hormone that boosts both your libidos.

- **Say no nicely** Reject sex, *not* your partner, by making it clear you're not upset just because they want sex when you don't.

- **Take responsibility for your libido** Don't expect your partner to turn you on, do it yourself! Make it your mission to pinpoint what gets you in the mood for sex, then do more of it.

- **Sort out any body image issues** The better you feel about your body, the more you enjoy sex.

- **Sort out any family inheritances** Don't really like being touched, sexually or otherwise? Bet your family aren't touchy-feely either. I suspect when you were forced to touch as a family (kisses on birthdays, hugs goodbye) it was all a bit tense and awkward with bodies as stiff as ironing boards and people letting go of each other the second they could. If you're lucky, you grew up in a family where love is expressed through touch. If you weren't so lucky and your family didn't express love through touching, you haven't learned to link touching with love, let alone the next step, sexual pleasure. Sometimes, simply being aware of this can help you overcome the problem, some may need a little nudge along with the help of a good therapist, counselor, or a particularly wise friend.

- **Let your imagination loose** Don't be ashamed of your fantasies, and refuse to feel guilty if having sex with someone other than your partner is one of them. Being unfaithful in reality isn't alright but it's OK to do it in your head. Really.

- **Use lubricant to help you get aroused** If you're not aroused, you're probably also dry. Which means anything your partner does feels half as pleasurable as it should – and you feel self-conscious about it. Next time, add lubrication before you start having sex – reach in and place a big glob high inside the vagina and let the heat of your body and his fingers draw it downward. The added moisture not only makes everything feel better and you sexier, you stop worrying that your partner thinks you're not turned on and instead focus on what he is doing to turn you on.

- **Meet halfway** If you don't want intercourse, what about oral sex? If you don't want oral sex or any sex yourself, do you mind pleasuring them? At the very least, you can and should be able to offer the physical intimacy of a cuddle.

- **Focus on sex, don't avoid it** If you're constantly being hassled for it, sex is often the last thing you want to watch or read about. Low libido people often avert their eyes when they see nudity, a sexy scene on TV or in the movies, or flip the page if they hit a story in the newspapers or glossies. Don't. Stop feeling guilty for saying no and make yourself open to the positives of sex. It's just as easy to think yourself into sex as it is to talk yourself out of it.

- **Experiment with masturbation** For most people, the more they masturbate, the more their body gets used to having orgasms and the higher their libido. For others, it depletes what little urge they had. What works for you?

- **Know what you want**…and need to be satisfied sexually. And I'm talking both in and out of bed. If you need to relax first, don't be scared to ask for a massage. Or for them to do the dishes while you take a bath or shower.

- **Give sex a high priority in your life** If you're avoiding it or not interested, chances are it's the last thing you do, last thing at night. Well – Gosh! – funnily enough, even high sex drive people sometimes wonder if it's worth the effort when they're exhausted after a long day at work. Try sex before you start dinner and switch the TV on. Or if you really are too stressed during the week, have breakfast in bed on the weekends and have sex then.
- **Initiate sex, even if you're acting** If you've got a high sex drive and are always the one asking your partner for sex, you tend to think of yourself as the "sexy" person and the one who wants it less as the "less sexy" person. Initiating sex is a turn-on. It puts you in the sexual power position – and that alone can often kick-start a lazy libido. So if you're the "less sexy"'one, start something. Even if the resulting sex isn't that wonderful, your partner will be thrilled to bits that you're at least trying or, if they refused, you've gotten a taste of what it's like to be in their shoes.
- **Get your body clocks in sync** Is it really a case of mismatched libidos or a morning person matched with a nighttime one? Take turns on the time of day you make love. And try sex mid-morning and mid-afternoon.
- **Sex does NOT equal intercourse** Give each other orgasms through oral sex, or hand stimulation. Make sure sex doesn't always end with intercourse. Plenty of women especially don't orgasm through intercourse alone, so tend to find penetrative sex quite boring. The easier it is for you to orgasm, the higher your sex drive. And vice versa. Experiment with oral and manual techniques until you've explored all orgasm opportunities.

Reasons why you're not frothing at the mouth

Physical
- Exhaustion and stress
- Poor general health or chronic illness
- Excessive alcohol or drug abuse
- A reaction to medication or to recreational drugs
- Depression
- Low hormone levels
- Menopause, periods, and pregnancy all alter levels of desire
- Pelvic surgery (like hysterectomy) that has deadened nerve endings in the genital region
- No chemistry with partner

Emotional
- Relationships problems: feeling frustrated, angry, or resentful toward your partner or feeling guilty, sad, or ashamed about something you've done to them
- Low self-esteem or, more specifically low sexual self-esteem
- A bad lover: zero technique eventually leads to zero desire
- Bad body image and a lack of confidence as a result
- Poor sex education
- A traumatic earlier sexual experience or a history of unsatisfactory sex
- A strict religious upbringing that may have taught you sex is "bad" and other negative attitudes towards sex
- Communication problems that stop you telling your partner what triggers you need to tip you over the orgasm edge
- Lack of trust
- Tension – unresolved relationship conflicts, resulting in one or both of you withholding sex as a punishment

- **Don't relax while you're having sex!** Instead, focus on the erotic sensations you're feeling. Tighten the muscles of your thighs, bottom, lower stomach, and your pelvic floor muscles to help trigger an orgasmic reflex. Stay in the here and now. Try to tune out work worries, kids, bills, bad bosses. A stressed person is not a sexy person and everyday life is not erotic.

Initiating sex is a turn-on. It puts you in the sexual power position – and that alone can often kick-start a lazy libido.

- **Set up a craving cycle** It's a bit like the sugar craving you get when you sneak out for chocolate mid-afternoon. Your body learns to ask for what feels good. Without wanting to point out the obvious, orgasms feel good. Your body – quite logically – says "more please" and sulks if you don't obey by developing either psychological or physical cravings when denied its high. The more sex you have, the more you want. Furthermore, let's not forget that the emotional intimacy gained by physical intimacy can make it worth the effort. Have good sex and you're constantly reminded of all the physical and emotional pluses.
- **Put yourself on a sex initiation program** If you never initiate sex, this is particularly helpful. During the sexual initiation program, your partner remains "passive" when you initiate sexual contact. Make it clear that they're not to take it further: simply accept and enjoy what you're doing to them. It's important you spell this out to them or they'll naturally take over. They also need to give you permission to stop when you want. Lots of low libido people are too scared to start something, in case they don't want to follow through, so avoid even kissing their partner because they know they'll be badgered for sex when all they wanted was to cuddle. I've given a simple example of the program from the female perspective, reverse sexes for the male. The idea is to get you to relish being the one in charge rather than relying on them to do everything for you:
  Day one: You give him a sexy shoulder massage while he's watching TV.
  Day two: Add in a good long sexy smooch.
  Day three: Kiss him while putting his hands on your breasts. Encourage him to fondle them.
  Day four: Cuddle him from behind and feel and fondle his penis through his pants.
  Day five: You remove your own undies and ask him to give you oral sex.
  Day six: You remove his pants and give him oral sex
  Day seven: Seduce him completely, starting by kissing and ending with you getting on top and lowering yourself onto his penis.

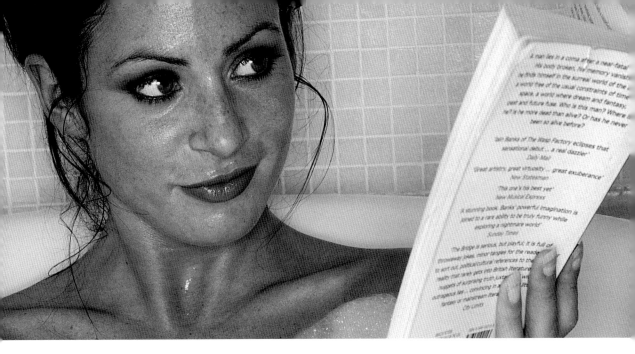

THE FIX-ITS: YOU WANT IT MORE THAN THEY DO

- **Don't hassle, masturbate** Take the edge off by having solo sex.
- **Redirect your energy** Shift the focus from your sex life to your relationship. Be affectionate and make it abundantly, blatantly clear you don't just want them for sex.
- **Make sure it's sex you're hungry for** Don't use sex as a replacement for intimacy, affection, sleep, or as a stress-reduction device.
- **Accept that "no" means no** And do it graciously.
- **Agree to let them take the exit route** If your partner agrees to give it a try to see if they can become aroused, let them exit if they want to. If they know they can stop at any stage, they'll be more likely to give it a try. If they do stop early, have a solo orgasm.
- **Don't take more than you need** Don't demand a smorgasbord of sexual delights when a snack would take away the hunger pains.
- **Create optimum sexual satisfaction conditions** Know what turns your partner on and off. If oral sex does it for them, explore all possible options. Learn new tricks and tips and broaden your sexual repertoire as much as possible in this area.
- **Don't confuse being loved with being lusted after** Just because their tongue's not hanging out from merely looking at you, doesn't mean they love or desire you less than you do them. Your sexual response system works quicker, that's all.
- **Learn to love quickies** All sex sessions don't have to be marathons. Use loads of personal lubricant and make the most of whatever time you do have.
- **Try magnet therapy** A clear way to communicate when you want sex, taking the awkwardness and guesswork out of it. Put two magnets on the fridge – one each – which you both move to show how horny you're feeling. The higher the magnet, the more you feel like sex. This removes the pressure of trying to second guess and the "less sexy" person can take control a little.

What women worry about
(and really shouldn't)

I don't care if you can twist yourself into 96 sexual positions, quote from the *Kama Sutra,* and tie a knot in a cherry stem simply by using your tongue (OK, I'm impressed with the last one). The fact is, you're never going to cut it as a sexpert if you spend most of your time in bed stressing rather than sighing.

THEIR BODIES

"She hates side-by-side sex because it makes her stomach look fat. She won't get on top because she's worried her breasts will look funny. She won't even go to the bathroom unless I promise not to look at her butt. Why won't she believe that I love her body as it is? I don't see these supposed faults," says my friend Ross. Most women are paranoid about their bodies and it's not just our self-esteem that takes a miserable dive every time we succumb to the "I bet my butt looks big" thing. A bad body image has a direct effect on our ability to enjoy sex. A billion studies have shown body self-conscious women are more timid and less likely to initiate sex, try new positions, or talk about their needs than women who are happy with their butt – I mean their lot. The truth is, men don't look at it and think "cottage cheese," they think "let me get my hands on that." In my experience, there's just one thing that freaks men out when you're getting naked: those cleavage-boosting things we now all stuff in our bras, which look like raw chicken fillets. You've got to admit you'd be alarmed if he plucked one out of his pants!

SUPERSEX SOLUTION Ideally, I'd love to just say "It's your inner beauty that's important, not your inner thighs," but I know you'll just say "That's crap!" and flip the page. How about "If you're the only naked woman in the room, he'll think you're beautiful"? Oh all right, here's something for the rest of you.

- **Light right** Standard lighting (from above) doesn't do anyone any favors. The most flattering: low-level. Try putting glass-encased scented candles on the floor.
- **Breasts** Get him to tie or handcuff you to the bedpost or bind your wrists above your head with a scarf. If your arms are stretched up or back, it pulls the bust tight and lifts even the saggiest of breasts.
- **Butt** Do it doggy-style. When you're on all fours, your butt looks smaller and firmer because the muscles and skin are stretched and taut.

- **Legs** If it's your calves that are the problem, pull on a pair of knee-high (better still thigh-high) boots and he'll hardly be questioning why. To lengthen legs, stockings and stilettos is another fail-safe killer combo.

- **Stomach** Missionary works but there is another alternative. Press your stomach flat against the bed/desk/kitchen counter top and ask him to penetrate from behind.

BEING TOO ENTHUSIASTIC/ EXPERIENCED

Ooops! Better not be too eager, he'll think I've done it before. And, God forbid, he'd think we were anything but virgins at the innocent age of…32. Like, honestly! Where did all this come from? Well, let's start with our family, the strongest influence of all on our sexual morals. Sixty-three percent of women say their attitudes toward sex were mainly shaped by good old Mom and Dad – and 66 percent of those said the messages they got made them feel bad about sex. They felt guilty for wanting to try it, and even guiltier when they did. If you had parents who told you sex was going to be something wonderful in your life and they gave you good, accurate information about it, you're pretty lucky. Parents aren't the only ones who help spread the "sex is something men will do anything to get" message. From a very young age, it's blatantly obvious you're meant to hold off "giving" a guy "what he wants" for as long as possible and if you do "give in" too soon, you're a bad girl. Lots of people who grow up with strict, religious parents get one message about sex: it's something wicked you shouldn't do. Even the most sheltered child knows what a "slut" is. Is it any wonder, even given the benefit of age and wisdom, that it's pretty hard to shake off all that stuff and enjoy sex later on without feeling guilty?

And the stuff that seems silly but actually isn't…

- **Will anything happen to me if I swallow my boyfriend's semen?** It's not harmful to your health since semen is mostly water and mucus (though there are traces of citric acid, salt, chloride, ammonia, vitamin C, calcium, carbon dioxide, and cholesterol: sperm is only one percent of ejaculate!). The only potential problem is a large one though – if he carries a sexually transmitted disease (STD), you may get it. Take your pick from the list of diseases that can be passed on this way (gonorrhea, chlamydia, hepatitis B, HIV). In fact, just wrapping your mouth around his penis puts you at risk of contracting herpes, human papillomavirus (genital warts), or syphilis, if they're present. Sorry if I've scared you so much you're racing to the STD clinic to test for all STDs, but these are the facts (and it won't kill you to have a few tests and might even save your fertility!). P.S. There is some good news – it's not fattening! There are a mere five calories in the amount of semen ejaculated.

- **Can you get pregnant without intercourse?** While it's very rare to become pregnant if you haven't had intercourse, it is possible. If you're excited and well-lubricated and he ejaculates on or very near the vaginal opening, there is a risk of pregancy. Similarly, the pitter-patter of tiny feet might not just be your cat padding down the hall if he has semen on his fingers and inserts them into your lubricated vagina. While we're on the subject, let's dismiss another popular myth: that you can't conceive during your period. You can. Sperm can live up to eight days in a woman's reproductive tract. This means a few still lurking around up there, waiting to pounce on an unsuspecting egg if ovulation occurs at that time.

SUPERSEX SOLUTION Actively challenge the thoughts and expose them for the complete and utter nonsense they are. Every time you think, "I'm bad for enjoying sex" think of the woman you most admire and substitute her name. "Sarah is bad for enjoying sex." How would she feel if you said it to her face? She'd think you were nuts! Better still, make that a *man* you admire. Makes you realize how silly and how hopelessly old-fashioned the whole concept is!

NOT HAVING AN ORGASM EVERY SINGLE TIME

Most men orgasm each time they have intercourse – unfortunately for us, the female response isn't as reliable or automatic. The mood we're in (fat/thin/bad hair/good hair day), how energetic we feel (Should I go to the store to buy some chocolate or get them to deliver it along with the video?), what's happening in our lives and relationships (He's being a bastard again), the amount and type of foreplay (Was that it?), and the amount we've drunk (I seem tobe havinngck ploblims having an horrgashm hunny): all these factors affect whether or not we climax. If you feel

Stop worrying about **being "slutty"** and start worrying about **being boring.**

secretly guilty about sex, it's unlikely you'll be relaxed enough to orgasm. Sometimes an infection or other gynecological reason is to blame. But more often than not it's not enough foreplay, the wrong type, or an ineffective foreplay technique – sometimes a terrible combination of all three.

SUPERSEX SOLUTION Step 1: Read a few (more) good sex books and educate yourself on your body's sexual responses. Don't just to figure out how to bring your body to the brink, but also work on how you reassure yourself that it isn't "you" but the way our bodies are built that stops us from having effortless orgasms. (Thanks God, we owe you one.) Step 2: If you're not doing it already, start masturbating – and pay attention. What exactly are you doing with your fingers to make yourself climax: think speed, technique, pressure, what's your other hand doing? Any other crucial factors (time of day, light, music, privacy factors)? If you're relying on vibrotherapy for your solo climaxes, then you're not doing yourself or your partner any favors. He can replicate what you do with your fingers, but short of plugging himself into the nearest socket, a vibrator is a hard act to follow. Step 3: (and please tell me you've been paying attention and have gotten this message already) show or tell him what works. The final stage: Up your chances of orgasming while he's inside you, by using something that therapists call "the bridge maneuver" (see p.111): he stimulates your clitoris with his fingers while you have intercourse.

NOT WANTING SEX AS MUCH AS HE DOES

"It's been the same with every girlfriend I've ever had. They're all over you in the beginning but stop wanting it at all once you've been together for awhile." The immortal words of my friend Michael, muttered at some stage by every other male on planet Earth. The claim: We only seem to like sex at the beginning. Once the relationship is serious, we lose interest. Some guys think it means we're just not interested in sex at all. We fake it in the beginning until we've "got him," then drop the act. Apart from a few exceptions (Julie Andrews and a very strange girl I met on a plane once), I think there's a far less sinister and more logical explanation. Women get bored with sex if it becomes predictable. And if we're bored, it's hard to have an orgasm

Not sure if **you're being a prude?** Depends on what he's asking for. If it's sex with the light on, you're a prude. If it's **sex with the next-door neighbors,** you're not.

because we need a lot more stimulation than a man does to topple us over the edge. If we're unlikely to experience an earth-shattering treat after all that effort, why bother? I admit, it's not the healthiest of attitudes, but it is an understandable reaction.

SUPERSEX SOLUTION Stop sex from becoming routine by trying new things. And stop worrying about being "slutty" and start worrying about being boring. Ask him to write down 10 new things he'd love to try but is too scared to ask. Do the same; then swap lists. Check out those things you think would be worth a whirl. Not sure if you're being a prude? Depends on what he's asking for. If it's sex with the light on, you're a prude. If it's sex with the next-door neighbors, you're not. Experimentation is healthy and any reasonable request should at least be considered, although feel free to say no. Ask yourself: Will it have an adverse physical effect on my body? Will it have an effect on me emotionally? Will I feel resentful afterward? Most important, am I doing it to stop my partner from leaving me? If the answers are "yes," forget it – and him. If you skate through these without coming up with a good reason for not trying it, agree to try it once.

Ant meets elephant
What to do if things don't fit

We all worry too much about the size of our parts. About 85 percent of men think penis size is important to women; most women think men crave someone with the vaginal muscles of a Thai sex worker. In reality there's really only one instance when a small penis or a large vagina cause problems: when the owner is so paranoid and insecure about it, that they're constantly apologizing, seeking reassurance, and becoming inhibited in bed. Now that really is boring.

In an ironic twist of fate, I had the bizarre experience of sleeping with the man with the smallest penis in the world and the man with the biggest penis in the world right after one other. The first guy I went out with for a year (and, oh all right, hold four pens together for the width, then halve them for the length – yes, that small) and he turned out to be so wonderfully good at oral, sex that I seriously wouldn't have cared if he hadn't had a penis at all.

A few months after we broke up, I dated Mr. Big. We slept together – as in shared a bed – about a week into the relationship. He had his PJ bottoms on and I had on the top, which was all nice and cozy until I woke to feel this thing prodding me in the back. Thinking "No, that can't possibly be it because…well, it just can't be," I drifted off again. Silly girl. I should have run while I had the chance. Several dinners later and it was D-Day. I gulped, he reached under the bed to produce an economy-size, pump-pack of lubricant and an extra-large condom that the entire US army could have camped inside. Then he unceremoniously unzipped his pants to unleash The Beast. He slapped on more lubricant than a brothel would use in a week, stared me in the eye, and said (and I'm not joking), "Climb on board, baby." He wasn't joking either. I considered using a stepladder but instead tried to lower myself onto him, feeling like Jack about to be impaled on the beanstalk. It was just awful! He was the width of a soda can. It turned out that his ego was (almost) as big as his penis. Not surprising, then, it was the worst sex I have ever had.

And the moral of the story is…well, it's pretty obvious, really. Penis size does not equal sexual prowess. Luckily, a sexual mismatch like mine doesn't mean you're doomed forever. Lopsided love isn't a problem if it's confined purely to the genital area. So whether Cupid's aimed his arrow to link a small penis with a large vagina or matched petite with jumbo the other way around, it all evens out in the long run. Here's how…

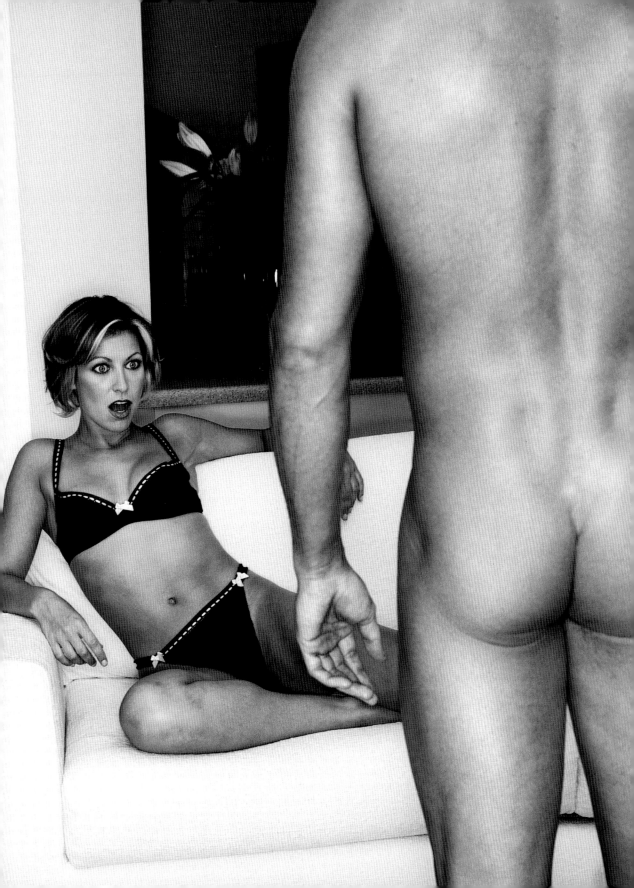

In society's eyes, a big penis is something to boast about and sometimes the owner thinks that's enough on its own to turn women on. So he doesn't bother developing any foreplay skills and becomes very penetration focused by tending to think of sex as intercourse only. I'm not saying all well-endowed men are like this, but some do get a little carried away with the I've-got-a-big-one thing. The fact is that while whopping great penises may impress other men, they tend to freak women out.

The organ most important to female sexual arousal is the clitoris, not the vagina, and it's stimulated by hands and tongues, not by a thrusting penis. Further evidence: a vagina can only feel stimulation in

He produced an **economy-size** pack of lubricant and an **extra-large condom** that the **entire US army** could have camped inside.

the one or two inches nearest the vaginal opening – and that's it. ALL of the nerve endings in the vagina are located at the mouth of the vagina. This is to prevent (even more excruciating) pain during childbirth. So assuming that your penis is longer than two inches (see below if it's not), it's more than adequate. The rest of the vagina receives little sensation from the penis, no matter how big it is. You're worried about width not length? Width doesn't matter either since the vagina stretches only enough to accommodate the penis. The fact is, even if you are a genital mismatch, it should be blatantly obvious from reading all this that Mother Nature's already thought of the solution. Lecture over. Now here's some practical advice that should clear up any residual problems!

BIG PENIS/SMALL VAGINA:
She should:
- Make sure you're fully aroused before he penetrates, so that the vagina expands and lubricates. Spend lots of time on foreplay so that you can accommodate him.
- Push down with your vaginal muscles while he's penetrating.
- Comfort yourself with logic: your vaginal muscles are elastic enough to take the biggest penis – after all, you can deliver a baby from the same place!
- Get him to try massaging the entrance of your vagina with his fingers, using a water-based lubricant, for several minutes before intercourse.

He should:
- Squeeze that tube of lube! – even if she's wet to start with.
- Penetrate slowly, and stop each step of the way so that your bodies become accustomed to each other. Let her control the insertion.
- Try penetrating from different angles to see which feels comfortable. If you're really big, she might not want full penetration. Keep thrusting shallow and gentle.
- Have intercourse just before she's about to have an orgasm from oral sex or manual masturbation so that she's as lubricated and expanded as possible.

Prime positions

- Choose positions that don't allow deep penetration: her-on-top, so she can control the depth of his thrusts; or side-by-side facing each other, her resting her upper leg over his hips. Or missionary with a twist: she tightly closes her legs to minimize access as he thrusts – this not only helps control the depth of penetration, but it also feels better for him.

SMALL PENIS/BIG VAGINA

She should:

- Do kegel exercises (see p.106).
- Have lots of nonpenetrative orgasms first. Don't make intercourse the main event.

He should:

- Get the right attitude. Accept the insignificance of the situation.
- Put two pillows beneath her butt when she's underneath. Put your legs on either side of hers, instead of getting her to open hers wide.

Prime positions

- She lies on her back and wraps her legs over his shoulders, narrowing the vaginal canal and allowing him deep access, or she kneels on all fours and he penetrates from behind. Or she lies on her back and brings her knees up to her chest. He penetrates from on top with her feet resting on his shoulders.

OTHER TRICKS FOR LOPSIDED LOVERS...

His penis is too thin? She lies face down, he enters from behind while she squeezes her legs together. He's too tall? She jumps on top. He's too short? Find uneven ground: he stands while she sits on the edge of a table or chair then she straddles his hips while holding his shoulders. He's a heavyweight? Again, she jumps on top, or he sits in a chair while she straddles him.

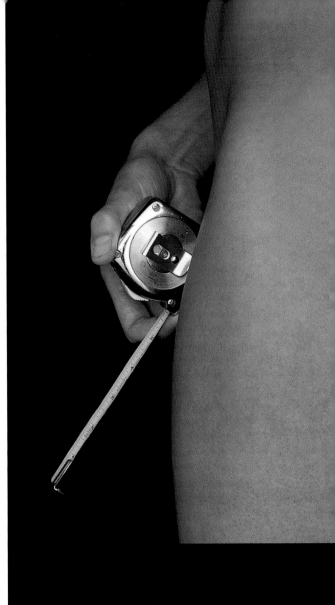

While whopping great penises may impress other men, they tend to **freak women out.**

"This is really embarrassing but..."
Your most humiliating sex questions answered

Some sex secrets we'll cheerfully share over the back fence with a neighbor ("Don't you think X — insert name of latest heartthrob — is sex on legs?"). Others we spill, along with the wine, at a good friend's dinner party ("In fact, put X in front of me in real life and there's no telling what I'd do. Sorry, honey.") And then there are those we don't dare share with anyone ("and not only are they wearing a bright purple raincoat but my same-sex primary school teacher's there as well. Like what does THAT mean??!!").

Well, it's those secrets that this chapter is all about. Those nagging, albeit silly, sexual fears that spin around and around our heads at 3am while the rest of the world sleeps. We all have them – but we don't always have the answers. Well, now you do! Because I spend each and every day writing or talking about sex, I've had just about every sex question there is come across my desk. So to speak. Here's a selection of the most common (and quirky): hopefully they'll inform as well as amuse…

Can too much sex make my vagina too loose?

No. But not enough sex can. Our vaginas are more a case of "use it or lose it" (muscle tone, that is). Popping out babies and aging cause your pelvic floor muscles to loosen and atrophy. Regular sex helps tone them and keep your vagina tighter. Single right now? Another great way to keep them in tiptop shape is to do kegel exercises. Kegels involve contracting and relaxing your PC (pubococcygeus) muscle. It's the same muscle you use to keep from peeing when there's no bathroom in sight. Identify the muscle then squeeze and hold it for a few seconds, release, then squeeze again. Work up to around 150 repetitions per day (for more information see p.106).

I'm paranoid that my vagina smells and convinced my boyfriend's far too polite to tell me if it does. How do I know for sure?

Listen, honey, if he's in it for the long haul, no one's that polite. Don't believe me? Let's apply some logic. Does he happily initiate oral sex or do you have to lure him with luscious treats (like the fries off your plate or baseball tickets) before he'd dream of venturing downward? If it's the latter, then ask him if there's a problem. Say "You don't seem that eager to give me oral sex. Is there a problem? Do I smell or something? I'd rather you told me, so I can fix it." If he says,

"Now that you mention it…", make an appointment to see your doctor/gynecologist asap. You could have a yeast infection (easily cured) or a ghastly bacterial upset called *gardnerella vaginalis*, which produces a charming fishy odor. A healthy vagina smells slightly acidic but it's certainly not unpleasant.

He's given you the all-clear? Stop panicking and stay fresh by bathing regularly, using nonscented soap, wearing cotton underwear, and giving feminine "hygiene" products a wide berth. Not only do they irritate the vagina and kill off good bacteria, but they also taste awful (if you want to taste just how awful then try licking your boyfriend's armpit after *he's* applied deodorant!).

Can you get pregnant from oral sex?

No. Sperm are clever little devils and can wriggle their way past all kinds of obstacles, but they haven't yet figured out how to dodge major organs like the heart and lungs to get to where they can fertilize an egg.

During intercourse my testicles disappear! Should I be worried?

Apparently, it can be a little alarming the first time you notice it but, trust me, nothing funky is happening. The testicles retract into the body because muscles in the area pull the scrotum toward the body during sex. It's good old Mother Nature's way of trying to keep things at the right temperature. She's also being protective and keeping them out the way of possible knocks during a particularly enthusiastic bout of intercourse. Rescue them afterward by gently pulling them down again. But if they tend to stay up there for long periods, see a doctor – it could affect your fertility because it's too hot for sperm to survive up there.

I'm always reading about sperm "shooting" out, but mine just oozes. Is this a problem?

Sperm is ejaculated through the opening in the head of the penis by the muscle spasm of orgasm. The force at which it is projected depends on the force of the muscle contractions: the more powerful they are, the farther the sperm "shoots." Why some men could aim for China and probably get there and others just "ooze," as you put it, is simply because we're individuals. Your penile muscle strength is like all the other muscles in your body – it varies according to genes and fitness level (which is how often you use them). Another factor is the consistency of your semen, affected by diet, health, and how often you ejaculate. The thinner the semen, the farther it will spurt.

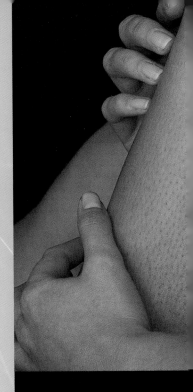

Sperm are clever little devils and can wriggle their way past **all kinds of obstacles,** but they haven't yet figured out how to **dodge major organs**.

Why do men get erections when they sleep? My girlfriend gives me a really hard time about this.

Well it's obviously because you're all obsessed sex maniacs who, even in slumber, only have one thing on your minds. Or that's what some women (namely your girlfriend) think. The truth is that while you may be nocturnally fantasizing about strawberry jam and Pamela Anderson's breasts, the cause is more likely to be a biological one, because sleep erections seem unaffected by the frequency, amount, or quality of sex you're having. Most men have several erections per night during the REM (Rapid Eye Movement) stage of sleep. Research shows that bursts of different types of brainwaves occur during REM periods, causing your pulse and breathing to race and your eyes to zigzag crazily (hence the name). All these reactions suggest that the nervous system is being aroused, which could easily trigger a reflex erection. So go ahead: stun her with science. And while you're at it, tell her she's as guilty of nighttime arousal as you are. By monitoring the genitals during sleep, researchers have found the same kind of arousal responses – the vagina expanding and lubricating – in women as well. You just can't see what she's up to!

The male G-spot (the prostate gland) is also located in **this hot spot.** If your partner strokes or presses it with a downward movement, I expect you'll get **a pleasant surprise.**

My boyfriend is a slave to computer games and most of them seem to involve big-breasted, long-legged Barbie-with-a-libido-type women. It's really starting to annoy me. Should I be threatened?

Young boys all over the world unwrapped the computer game *Lara Croft: Tomb Raider* for Christmas, only to have it wrestled from their seven-year-old fingers within minutes by Dad. Dad then spent days – hell, months! – with his fingers glued to the keypad and couldn't have cared less if wife/sister/mother/father/boss were kidnapped, captured, and tortured while he was absorbed in the game. Yes, the women in computer games may look like Scandinavian stewardesses who've taken one too many visits to the plastic surgeon, but check out Aladdin from your niece's Disney video collection and you'll see that it all evens out. Besides, if you plan on censoring overidealized cartoon or computer body images, we might as well just go back to playing tic-tac-toe! Truly, this is just another example of how men (quite healthily, I think) can separate fantasy sex from reality sex. Lusting after a cyberchick isn't sinister or abnormal, it's just damn good fun – a harmless escape from dreary old real life. Assuming that's all he's escaping from and it's not from you or your relationship, I wouldn't worry.

You know the thing about "Is it in yet?" Well, sometimes I really feel like asking that question of my boyfriend. I can feel him penetrate but that's about it!

It's interesting that you don't comment on the size of your boyfriend's penis. Because that's the obvious question, isn't it: is he extremely small? If he is dramatically undersized, then there's your answer. If he's close to "normal" size, other factors are at play. I don't think that anyone would deny (men or women) that the first thrust is undeniably the best because that's the thrust you feel the most. Once thrusting continues, you become desensitized to the sensation. Your vagina gets tired and the muscles stop clenching his penis and it all (sorry guys) gets a little boring for that very reason: you don't feel much. Fix it by experimenting with different positions that alter the angle of the vagina. Try it with him thrusting from behind and keep your legs closer together, rather than wide apart, in any position. Put one or two pillows under your bottom while he's on top. Kegel exercises (see question 1) will also help. P.S. While we're on the subject of size, here's some trivia for you – half his penis is internal. It reaches deep inside the body, all the way to the pelvic bone!

Does he happily initiate **oral sex** or do you have to lure him with luscious treats – like the fries off your plate or **baseball tickets –** before he'd dream of **venturing downward?**

If a guy (that's me) is really into anal stimulation, does this mean I'm secretly gay?

No. But the whole "Does this mean I'm gay?/This is naughty/I really shouldn't be doing this" thing is all part of what makes it exciting. Add a huge helping of supersensitive nerve endings in that area to the formula and you begin to understand why bottom play is bliss for lots of people (both sexes, I might add). There's another reason why you, as a guy, enjoy being stimulated: The male G-spot (the prostate gland) is also located in this hot spot. It's on the front wall of the rectum and is a firm, walnut-sized mass. If your partner strokes it or presses it with a downward movement, I expect you'll get a pleasant surprise.

I've got big labia lips and am very embarrassed about it. It's stopping me from experimenting with sex because my vagina is so ugly.

The lips of the vagina come in many different colors, shapes, thicknesses, and combinations of all of the above. The trouble is, lots of women don't realize this, because it's not often we get to see women with their legs wide open (and nor, I imagine, would most of us want to).

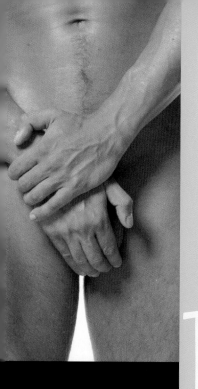

So we're forced to compare ours to those featured in any sex books we can get our hands on (line drawings which are so simplified, they're like a paint-by-numbers version of the real thing), or worse, in girlie magazines (where they've been air-brushed and "prettied" up via computer). If you could have a look at a full range of vaginas, you would soon see how yours isn't that different from the norm after all. Unfortunately, you're just going to have to trust me on this one. As for this influencing whether or not someone falls for you… Puhleeze! It doesn't matter what your labia lips look like, it's your attitude that matters. Stop worrying about something so unimportant. I have my hand on my heart when I say I'm one hundred percent sure no man is going to refuse to have sex with you because of this.

I've just started a relationship with the sexiest girl in the world. And that's basically the problem. I get so excited just looking at her naked, I orgasm before I've even touched her. Obviously, I'm not satisfying her, which means – just as obviously – that she's about to dump me unless I do something fast.

Several things are working against you – and only the last one's a problem: 1. You've snagged a Liz Hurley lookalike; 2. You're incredibly excited by her; 3. Because of the first two, you've got a problem with premature ejaculation. Which is perfectly understandable given the first two circumstances, don't you think? The problem will fix itself over time, but in the meantime you can help by doing the following: masturbate more while practicing holding off (count backward from 500); masturbate just before seeing her (it takes the edge off and you'll have more control after the first orgasm). Use distraction techniques: don't watch her get undressed, don't look at her naked body, close your eyes, and mentally compose your résumé instead (I know, I'm taking the fun out of it but it's only temporary). Finally, remove the pressure from yourself by ignoring it if you do orgasm too soon. Simply say, "Ooops! Too turned on again. Why don't I pleasure you until I'm ready for round two?" Move down to use your tongue or hands and I can't honestly see her having any complaints whatsoever.

Which feels better for her – a short, fat penis or a long, thin one?

That depends on whether her name is Mary, Martha, Marge, or Madge. In other words, it all depends on how she's made. Vaginas come in different varieties. If she's got a sensitive cervix or low-slung ovaries, then a long penis that reaches high in the upper vagina might cause pain rather than pleasure. If her vagina is wide, a short, fatter penis might make her feel more "filled up." Whatever you've got, it's unlikely she'll ditch you because of it. People don't fall in love with body parts, but rather, with the person they belong to.

People don't **fall in love with body parts,** but rather, with the person they **belong to.**

What happens if I lose a condom inside me?

The good news is it won't get lost (so those fears of coughing it up in front of your boyfriend's mom are well…silly). To remove it, squat down, reach in with a finger and feel around the walls of your vagina. If you can't find it, your doctor can. And you might need a visit anyway because you're obviously at risk of pregnancy since the semen's disappeared up there along with the condom. (Your risk of contracting an STD increases as well, since the condom obviously hasn't done its job of being a barrier between you and your partner.) If you don't detect it immediately and it stays up there for a day or so, you could also be at risk of an infection.

My boyfriend wants me to lick his anus. My reaction was "Are you crazy? No way" but he insists that it's quite normal and that lots of people do it.

I'm not sure that lots of people do it, but it's certainly not rare. It's an oral-anal activity called "rimming." In plain English, it's as you said: the act of licking someone's anus. As with licking anyone's parts, it sounds revolting until you're on the receiving end. The risk of hepatitis B and other infections is very

Picture a **clock dial around** the vagina. The top is noon. The lowest point is 6pm. When she starts **sighing and squirming**, chart the position and memorize it.

high though. You've got two options to protect against this. The first is to use a dental dam. It's a square of latex (rubber), slightly smaller than a tissue, which you put between your mouth and anyone's parts to protect you against infections. Unfortunately, they're not always readily available. The second option is for both of you to get yourselves down to that STD clinic and get blood and urine tests and swabs done so that you both get the all clear. You can't get an infection from someone who doesn't have one.

Just when I think I've got it all figured out and found the spot that makes her orgasm, she moves the goalposts. It seems to change each time. Is this true or am I imagining it?

No, you're not bonkers – it really does alter because things like mood, alcohol consumption, time of the month, etc., all affect the sensitivity of the clitoris. Happily, there is a technique that will help. Imagine the vagina as a clockface (bear with me, I'm not completely crazy). Go on, picture a clock dial surrounding the vagina. The top (near her pubic hair) is noon. The lowest point (near the vaginal opening) is 6pm. When she starts sighing and squirming, chart the position (2pm/3pm whatever) and memorize it. Not only do you avoid having to superglue your tongue to the spot that seems to be working that session (it's either that or leave a Hansel and Gretel breadcrumbs trail), but you've now also got the freedom to remove it to lick her breast, stomach, and upper inner thighs before (magically!) returning to the exact spot that was driving her wild with lust. If you're prepared to share your secret, she can use the clockface technique to direct you there in the first place.

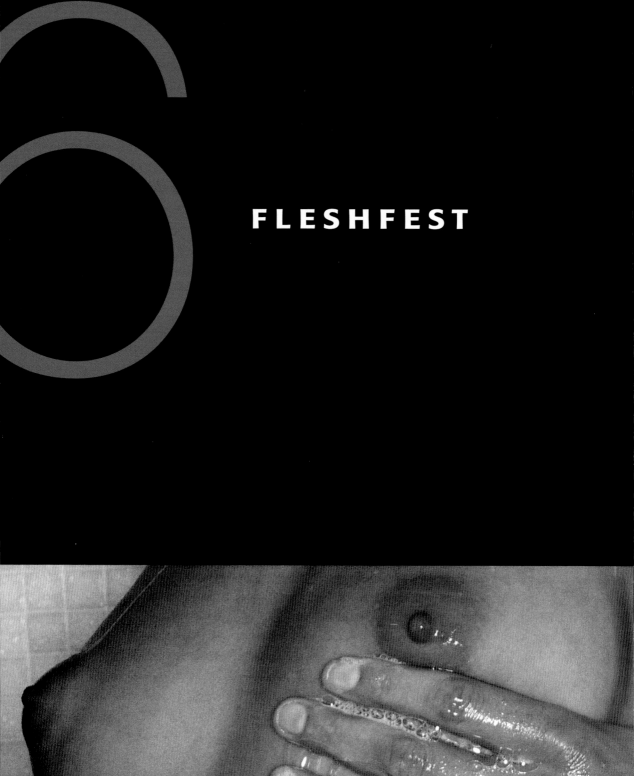

FLESHFEST

Why **being bad** makes you very, very good in bed, finding your own signature sex move, **the truth about aphrodisiacs**, and why **decidedly dirty** daydreams can save your **relationship**.

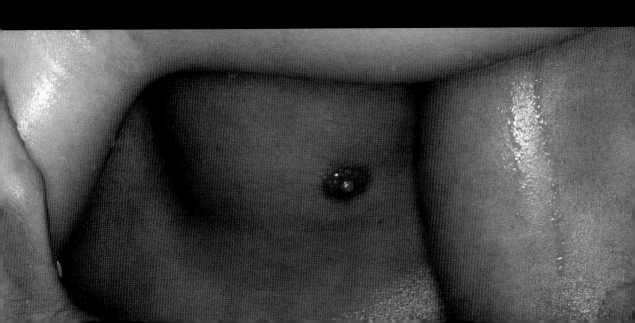

Sexual chemistry

Looking for a shortcut to take you to sexual nirvana? Join the club!

The search for a potion guaranteed to turn coy virginal girls into insatiable nymphomaniacs and men into sex machines capable of thrusting their way into the next millennium has been under way for centuries. Is alcohol really the libido-boosting lust elixir we think it is? Is Viagra all it's cracked up to be? The search for the ultimate sexperience continues…but the pot at the end of the rainbow may be emptier than you think.

Let me reveal something truly astonishing: great sex makes you feel good. Yes really. When we have great sex, endorphins – feel-good hormones – are released into our bodies. Not only do they make us feel all warm and fuzzy, but they also boost immune cells and create a feeling of well-being, providing a satisfying balance between stimulation and relaxation. The chemicals mainly responsible for this feeling are serotonin (the happy hormone) and dopamine (the cuddly hormone). Both are influenced by lifestyle and diet. Could it be then that sexual desire and pleasure is all down to what you put in your mouth? According to my friend Ian Marber (aka The Food Doctor), spicing up your sex life really could be as simple as changing what you put in your shopping cart…

A LITTLE GOES A LONG WAY…

Alcohol is probably the one substance that most would agree has positive aphrodisiac qualities. It relaxes us, reduces inhibitions, and lends courage to those usually too scared to make sexual advances. It's a case of a little of what you like being a good thing. The trouble is, having a lot of what you like can have the opposite effect. Many of the problems associated with psycho-pharmaceuticals are also true of alcohol. We let loose – but a little too much and in all senses. When we've got our "beer goggles" on we're much more likely to sleep with someone we wouldn't look at twice if we were sober. And we lose control of vital muscles. All those kegel exercises – when you religiously clenched and tightened the vagina – are rendered useless when you're sloshed. Dreams of squeezing him into nirvana by showing off superb muscle control evaporate quicker than the wine. Too much alcohol often leads to temporary impotence in men ("brewer's droop") and it makes both of you less sensitive, so it's often harder to reach orgasm. It all comes back to what I said earlier – and what you know is true (even if you don't really want to believe it): moderation is the key. A few glasses can pep up your performance; one drop too many and you've blown it.

EAT YOURSELF SEXY

The one thing guaranteed to have a positive effect on your sex life and therefore act as a true aphrodisiac is your diet. It stands to reason that the better your diet, the better you feel and the more energy and enthusiasm you'll have for sex (not to mention the obvious spin-off of looking better and so being happier to prance around the bedroom naked!) Nutritionists say eating certain foods, especially those high in specific nutrients, delivers a powerful boost to the libido. Women should aim to eat foods high in vitamins A and E, and boron (a trace element which helps production of sex hormones). Down loads of dairy products, oily fish, fruit, and all vegetables – particularly dark green ones. Men need supplies of zinc and vitamin B, which is found in shellfish, cheese, eggs, chicken, and turkey, bananas, potatoes, tuna, and avocados. Add imagination and anticipation to the grocery list and you'll both be contenders for the sexual Olympics.

AND FEEL FREE TO KID YOURSELF ABOUT THE FOLLOWING...

The Koreans and Chinese believe ginseng works wonders. Arabs favor cinnamon. Caviar, licorice, and chocolate have all been extolled at some point by Westerners. Some also believe that asparagus and rhinoceros horn will help him get an erection, while oysters and figs supposedly send her silly with desire. Some foods work because they are nutritionally important, others may have been chosen because of their similarities to the organ they're supposed to work their magic on – oysters and bananas being two obvious examples. In reality, it doesn't matter whether you feed them to each other or smear them all over your body, because the main benefit has to be that you feel it's doing you good, by boosting your sexual confidence.

Viagra

Despite popular perception, "V" isn't a real aphrodisiac because it only works in the presence of stimulation. It doesn't directly cause an erection but enhances the effects of nitric oxide, a chemical released when you're sexually stimulated. This relaxes the muscles, allowing increased blood flow into the penis, which itself leads to an erection. The drug then prevents the muscle walls of the blood-filled chambers of the penis from relaxing. Viagra is intended for use by men unable to achieve an erection but, of course, is being taken in handfuls by perfectly healthy men and women who hope for longer-lasting erections, highly sensitive and stimulated clitorises, and multiple orgasms.

Does it work for women?

A study done by US sex experts Jennifer and Laura Berman on the effects of Viagra on women found that although blood flow to the genitals increased, as with men, it did little in the way of arousal. In other words, their bodies were ready but it didn't follow that their minds were, just as an erection for him doesn't necessarily mean he wants to use it. If you do experiment, for goodness sake don't mix it with other drugs.

Side-effects

There are other downsides: headaches, hot flashes, and painful erections that last way longer than you want them to. A billion herbal spin-offs have infiltrated the market, as have "dream creams" (designed to increase blood flow to the vaginal area when rubbed on). Most herb-based preparations and creams are harmless if you follow instructions, so give them a whirl if you want, just don't expect miracles. And always remember that the true aphrodisiacs are your hands, mouth, tongue, and brain.

Game for anything
Why it's OK to be kinky

Shelve your inhibitions along with that book and get ready for a serious lust injection. Because this is where we go from mild to wild, with games for grown-ups: role-play, fantasies, and why it's OK to be "kinky." Yep! Not only is it acceptable, but it's preferable. People who fall into the dubious (desirable) "kinky" category are also more content with their sex lives, report the highest satisfaction with sex, have the most positive attitude toward it, have more orgasms, and suffer the least guilt and sexual difficulties. Did you really need permission? Didn't think so. Following are some starting points for...well, whatever you like really.

SEXUAL FANTASY

Sexperts used to argue that no one could become sexually aroused without being touched. Good luck finding anyone these days who doesn't agree that it's possible to arouse yourself using only your mind. Which is, by the way, great news for any couple in love who want to go the distance. Almost everyone has amused themselves on a subway/train/airplane by imagining what the stranger sitting opposite them would look like naked (on your lap, in your bed, over that convenient railing…). Sounds weird, I know, but this is actually fabulous news. While you might run out of new positions/ places/props/ techniques/ideas (in about 20 years), there's one thing that is limitless: your imagination. When the urge to play and stray strikes (and it will – it always does), fantasy and role-play are lovely ways of having the best of both worlds. By having the affair in your head, it boosts your sex life with your partner, giving it the saucy edge it needs to solve the sexual frustration of monogamy, without hurtful complications of a real-life affair. Does this mean most fantasies are better left in our imaginations? Quite frankly, yes! Most aren't meant to be brought to life (though there are exceptions). As my favorite advice columnist, Irma Kurtz of *Cosmo* puts it, most fantasies are, by definition, the free play of creative imagination: fiction, fakery, unreality. The whole point of them is that they're not real life. Take out the forbidden factor by making them real and you nearly always remove the appeal (not to mention get yourself into a whole lot of trouble). Many women have rape fantasies. This does not mean we want to be raped. Some men have same-sex fantasies. It does not necessarily make them gay. Some women get massively turned on imagining their partner having sex with another woman. In reality, he'd be castrated. I'm with Irma, when she says: if you're not one hundred percent convinced it'll be a huge success, don't force it to survive the transition to reality.

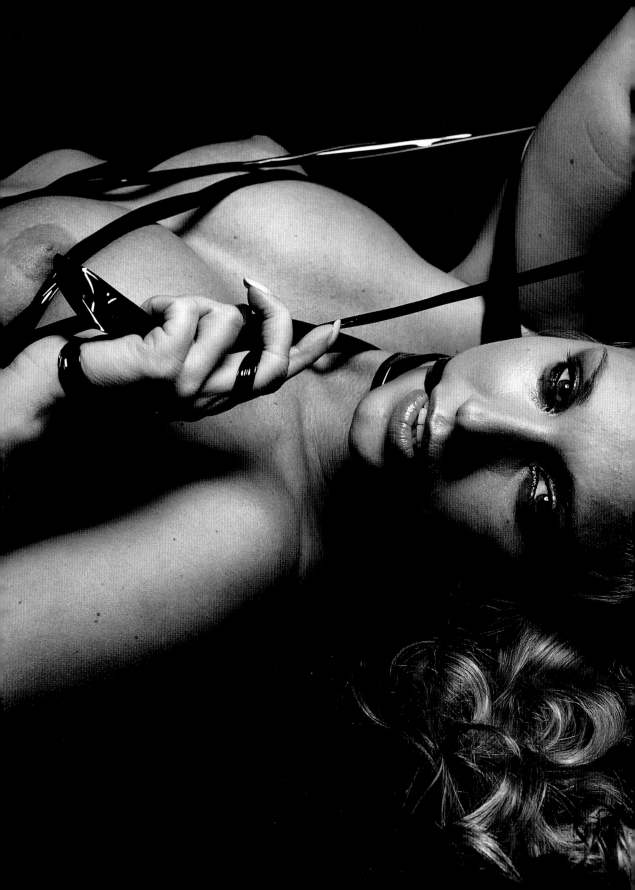

ROLE-PLAY

Ah-ha! Didn't I just say not to take fantasy through to reality? Well…yes. But I did say there were exceptions – and this is what I mean. It's one thing to sleep with the much-lusted-after local doctor or tell your partner you'd like to, but quite another to live out a sexy scenario where you're both playing roles. Here's the difference: "Honey, do you mind awfully if I call you Dr. Vincent during sex? You know, my gynecologist? Well, he's the guy who does my Pap smears and breast checks. And he's just soooooo dishy! Every time I have sex with you, I fantasize that you're him anyway, and if I could say 'Yes! Yes! Harder Dr. Vincent!' it would make it seem even more real. You don't mind, do you honey?…Honey?" Compare this to: "Honey, how about we play an X-rated version of doctors…and nurse?" Exactly.

Here's how to transform your risky fantasy into risqué role-play. First, get the general plot in your head. It's easier if you divide it into four parts: 1. Where/how you meet; 2. What happens when you do; 3. How does it all start happening; 4. What happens when it does (most detail here). Make it real by thinking about:

WHERE you should do it It's quite useful to role-play away from home (like on a dirty weekend) because it's much easier to pretend that you're someone else when you're not in familiar surroundings, which bring on familiar roles.

Do you LOOK the part? Role-play works best if you give your partner an instant visual jolt when they see you. Seeing you dressed as someone else, forces them to see you "anew" – as if they don't know you. (Especially effective if you've turned into best friends who sleep together, by the way.) What clothes do you need to buy/rent? Are there any other changes you need to make to your appearance to fit the part? Wigs are fantastic: they change your look so dramatically, you feel like a completely different person the instant you put them on. It's far easier to get into character as a blonde bimbo if you've got the long blonde hair to go with it. Or turn into a doctor when you've got the stethoscope. Masks also work, for the same reasons. They're something to hide behind.

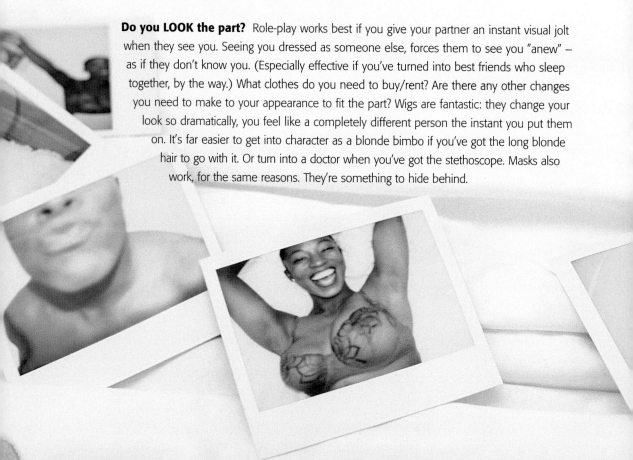

How to ACT? You've got the plot and the look, now work on the attitude! Get into character. Think of three adjectives you would use to describe the personality of the character you're playing. What about your partner? If you're in charge of the fantasy, give them specific instruction – or at least some clues – on how you want them to behave in their role. Below are two (ever-popular) scenarios to get those brain cells firing:

"Honey, do you mind awfully if **I call you Dr. Vincent during sex?** You know, my gynecologist?"

- **The sex worker** She wears super-revealing (OK, slutty) clothes under a big coat. You drop her off on a street corner (chosen carefully for obvious reasons). Park up the street and watch her, pretending she's a sex worker. Then cruise up, roll the window down, call her over, and ask how much. Get her to unbutton her coat and show you what you're getting for your hard-earned cash. Negotiate, then she gets in. On the way (home/somewhere remote) tell her what you want her to do; she'll tell you what she'll give you for the price. Keep everything cold/hard/impersonal (emphasis on hard).

- **Pick-me-up** Choose the type of venue you'd go to if you wanted to pick someone up (a bar?), then plant your partner there. Get him to strike a pose – as in, settle where he would if he were, in real life, single. Then, you make your move, i.e. blatantly pick him up for a one-night stand. Yes, you'll both want to laugh and whatever you say sounds contrived. But, hello! I bet a box of chocolates you both really did say that sort of stuff when you first met. You can play it as a repeat of your first night together or be two strangers who pass like ships in the night.

REVISIT the fantasy…instantly by deciding on a code word. If you were "Jane/Jake" during the role-play, saying "I bet Jane/Jake would love that" is your cue for both of you to go back into character.

.And when you've done all those, give these a whirl

Buy a case of his favorite wine and wrap 12 notes around the neck of each bottle, detailing things you're planning to do to him as you're sharing the wine.

Challenge her to a game of sexual scrabble. Follow the normal rules but all the words have to be connected to sex. Make sure you spell out deliberate messages about what you'd like to do to her once the game's over.

Let him play peeping Tom. Pretend to undress and masturbate as though you're alone but let him watch you.

Book a weekend at a sexy luxury hotel. Wrap up the brochure with a handwritten weekend itinerary of what you intend to do to her.

Write sexy notes and leave them in unexpected places. Like stuck on a bottle of beer in the fridge/on the bathroom mirror/in his wallet ("If you were here now, I'd be on my knees"). Confess your most erotic fantasy – and promise to do it.

Roll with it: *Cosmo's* come up with a winner with Vice-Dice: you need three to decide what you'll be doing sexually that night. Die one decides where (kitchen table, the car, in front of the window with lights on). Die two decides what (particular position, oral, masturbation). Die three decides what with (a blindfold, bondage, camera).

The way to keep anyone interested in anything is to do what's least expected. No matter how amazing a sexual maneuver, it'll be about as exciting as doing the dishes, if it's always delivered in the same way. Capture the spirit of unpredictability and you'll be the favorite for the Most Valued Lover Award.

BLINDFOLDS

…are excellent for helping to create the right atmosphere for role-play – particularly if you're rotten actors. They reduce embarrassment and increase awareness of physical sensations because you're closing off one sense, which highlights all the others. You can't anticipate what's in store next, so are forced to stay in a perpetual state of excitement. Poor thing.

The Shy Dominatrix Blindfold him, lead him into the bedroom, tie his hands behind his back, and get him to lie on the bed. Now, take him to the brink of orgasm and back again, time and time again. Kiss him. Rub your breasts against his chest, let him take a nipple in his mouth, then remove it (almost) immediately. Lower yourself over him for oral sex, let him smell you, then lift off again. Later, let him give a few licks, then get off (I know, it's hard). When he is, lower yourself over his throbbing manhood (Sorry but I had to get that phrase in somewhere) let him penetrate, then climb off almost immediately. Follow that with the best kissing he's ever had, but no body contact. Then go back and do it all again, but each bit for longer. When you've brought him to boiling point several times – at least three "almosts" – climb on top and let him climax.

SPANKING

One in 10 men fantasize about spanking a woman's bottom and one in 20 wishes she'd do it to him. The statistics for women aren't as clearcut, but it's certainly a popular fantasy.

Indulge her by…Pulling down her skirt/pants but leave them around her knees (part of the game is the humiliation), then bend her over your knee. Warm up the buttocks first by kneading them firmly, as though they're dough, throwing in a few light, playful slaps. Start to get firmer and heavier and play cheek to cheek, like her bottom is a set of drums. Vary your strokes so you're mixing light with quick, firm smacks. Alternate with teasing touches when you brush your fingers between her legs. If she seems to enjoy it, introduce props: the back of a hairbrush; the bottom of a pair of shoes; a wooden spoon. Always keep your spanks on the too light side rather than the too heavy and ask her to say "harder" to up the pressure.

BONDAGE

Being tied up and in control are mutually exclusive – hence the appeal to stressed-out business types who (statistically) relish bondage games and not having to be the boss. It's also appealing to women hung up on the Good-Girls-Don't issue: with the loss of control comes removal of responsibility, a gift that removes blame, guilt, and inhibition even quicker than it removes clothes. Others love it just because it's wicked (and you get to play dress-up).

How to transform yourself from Ms. Butter-Wouldn't-Melt-in-My-Mouth to Madame Lash

The look: ditch the lace for leather – preferably black or red. Chokers work well. Think tight and clingy rather than loose and flowing: lace-up boots and corsets, the higher and spikier the shoes, the better. *The personality:* start initiating sex more and taking more control. You get on top and stay there. Keep your top and bra on and if he tries to remove it, say "No!" forcefully and pin his hands down on either side of his head. Ride him mercilessly. *Action:* by now, he should be getting the drift of things. Use your (worn) stockings to tie his wrists behind his back. If he's not complaining at this point, he's yours to do with as you will…

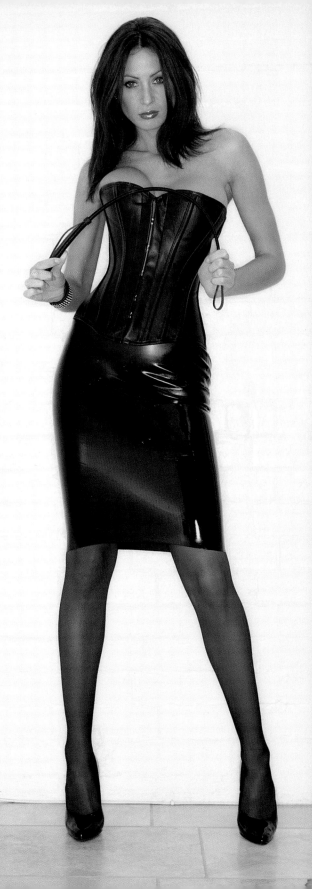

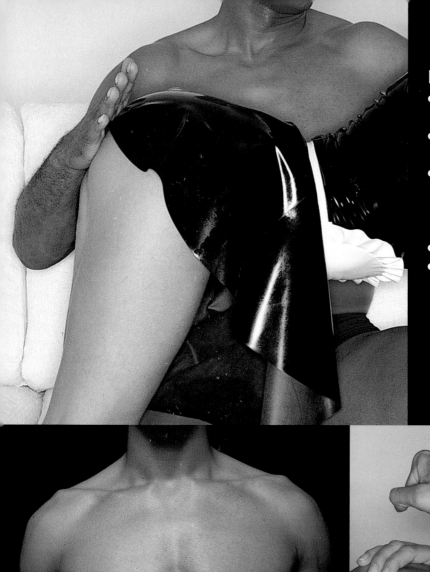

Kinky sex: the rules

- If trust is missing, it just isn't going to work.
- Set boundaries before you start. What's off-limits?
- Have a code word which means "stop." Make it nonsexual and easy to remember, like the name of a fruit or color.
- Don't be scared to laugh.
- Don't get too drunk beforehand. You'll lose perspective, the plot, and often your erection as well.

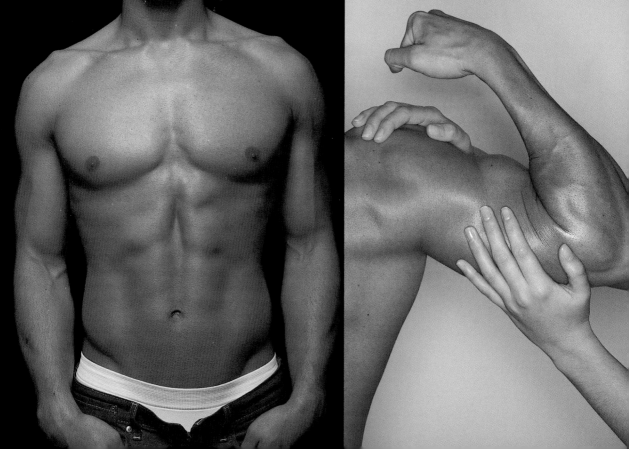

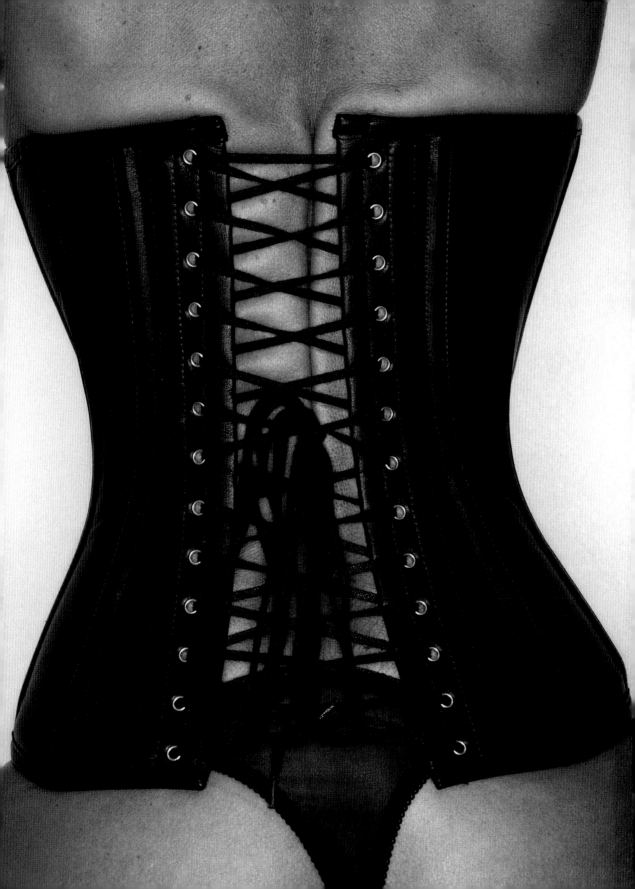

Wild women do...

...and bad girls finish first

Have you heard the news? There's a new breed of women out there and they're a bunch of shameless hussies! Selfish, self-absorbed – why, they're she-devils! Determined to destroy our sense of community/the American way/the family unit by putting off marriage and motherhood to concentrate on their own needs. Imagine! Daring to be independent rather than dependent. Slaves to a "me-first, others-later" ideology. Worshippers at the altar of self-gratification! I've even heard they have more than one lover at once! Zero inhibitions and libidos that rev faster than a Lamborghini. Sigh! Isn't it just *wonderful* being a woman in the 21st century?

FOUR-LETTER WORD

I turned on the TV in the UK the other night and saw some woman say, "It's quite obvious Robbie Williams [Britain's answer to Mark Wahlberg] would be a great lay – I mean, just look at him." On closer inspection, that woman turned out to be me. Quite frankly, it was recorded so long ago, I'd forgotten I'd done it – one of those let's-pick-fault-with-celebrities-because-we'd-all-like-to-be-them shows where "experts" like me say we wouldn't walk in their shoes for a million dollars (but secretly we'd pay them $100 for five minutes worth). Anyway, I was horrified. Why? Well, for a start, the lighting was awful and I looked about 150 years old (which blew my chances of Robbie calling the station for my phone number to prove the point, which was, after all, the whole point of doing the show in the first place). My second moment of mortification: "Everyone will think I'm right out there for saying that." I mean, I practically had my tongue on the floor like some sluuuuu…And then I stopped myself. Because not only do I hate the word and all its connotations, I thought "Oh what's wrong with it? It's a compliment and – it's true. He would be great in bed. Damn good in bed"…and proceeded to drift into some rather wicked Robbie fantasies that put me in a hell of a lot nicer place than squirming around imagining what my first-grade teacher now thinks of me. After all, who would I rather impress: the 70-year-old (and that was then) Mrs. Friar or the so-fresh-he-should-be-refrigerated Mr. Williams?

We're always talking about how women love bad boys (like Robbie and Mark). Well, wild women are just as appealing, for all the same reasons that we love a trashy video and a candy bar around the same size, or a whopping great G&T at the end of the world's worst work day. We all love doing

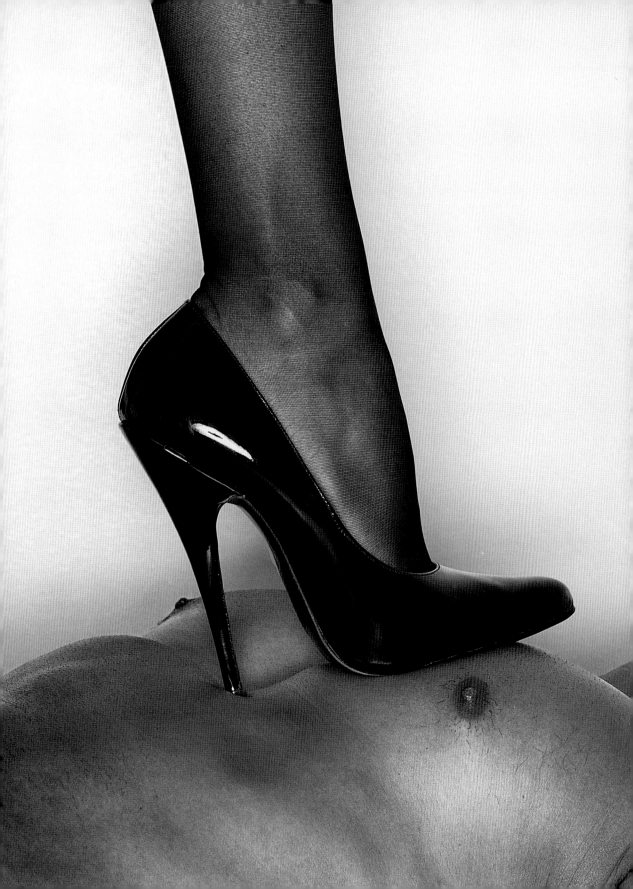

things that we shouldn't – and boys are as much a sucker for this as we are. Wild women aren't quite as easy to spot as bad boys. Apart from wicked thoughts and a slightly wanton attitude, I'm not quite sure what defines a bad girl. Sure, she'll flash a smile bigger than Julia Roberts' and maybe start twirling her hair with her little finger, while letting her gaze drop, just for a millisecond, downward. But apart from that…and maybe the wonderfully figure-hugging little black dress and the rather risqué thing she's doing with the straw in that cocktail, and…OK, whatever it is, you know it when you see it. And you also know anyone that delicious is not necessarily going to be the mother of your future children. But God, wouldn't it be wonderful if that fabulous body also housed a brain and even an ounce of humanity and vulnerability and…yikes! It does! So you try to be sensible and stop flirting. But the fact that you can't/shouldn't/won't makes it worse. Two drinks later you're frothing at the mouth. And…oh, just give in! You know you want to. Anyway, what was I saying about the difference between bad boys and wicked women? There is none. Which, given the appeal, is possibly why you might want to cash in on the whole thing…

She'll **flash a smile bigger than Julia Roberts'** and maybe start **twirling her hair with her little finger,** while letting her gaze drop, just for a millisecond, downward.

WANNA BE WILD? YOU'VE GOT TO…

- **Dress the part** By leaving something on like a great bra or high heels and a G-string. Think Victoria's Secret style rather than those awful black/red crotch- and nipple-less numbers. Open the bedside drawer of a wild woman and you'll also find panties that tie up on the side (for easy removal), a feather boa, some old scarves and stockings for tie-me-up games, chokers, satin French undies, black, white, and fishnet stockings, and every type of underwear possible, ranging from sporty and athletic to mere wisps of string so flimsy it's amazing they hold together. Wild women have lots of different sexual sides and dress to reflect them.

- **Talk the part** The turn-on of talking dirty is that (most) women aren't explicit about sex the rest of the time. So if you're the type who swears like a fishwife during PTA meetings, it's probably not going to surprise him particularly if you continue doing it in bed. The appeal harks back to the old "Madonna in the kitchen/whore in the bedroom" thing, so works best for wide-eyed wild girls who play pure and virginal in public and save their temptress-with-Tourette's-syndrome for behind closed doors.

- **Take control** You are mistress of the manor, he is the butler, so therefore must do anything you ask him to. "Get me a glass of wine." "Get me my bathrobe." "Run the bath." "Soap me up." You get the picture: the requests get dirtier the longer you play the game. He must say "Yes ma'am" after each request or he's banished to the kitchen to do the dishes and polish the silver.

- **Call the shots** Ban intercourse for the next five sessions so that you're forced to discover new ways to please each other. *First session:* you're only allowed to use your mouths, no hands allowed. *Second session:* hands only, no mouths or tongues. *Third session:* only allowed to stimulate lower half of body. *Fourth session:* only allowed to stimulate upper half of body. *Fifth session:* only intercourse allowed (and I bet it's the best lay you've had in ages!).

- **Have no shame** Take one of his hands in both of yours. Start by sucking his fingers, then run his hand over your neck, down over your breasts and your tummy, up your skirt to rub your clitoris through your panties. Don't let go at any point – his hand is a mere tool you're using to pleasure yourself.

If you're the type who swears like a fishwife during **PTA meetings**, it's probably not going to surprise him particularly if you **continue doing it in bed.**

- **Text tease** Let your fingers do the walking over that mobile phone keypad. "I got so hot thinking about us last night, I've just had to masturbate. My fingers are doing what I want yours to do to me tonight. I want you in my mouth." (Triple-check the number before you press the send key, it takes just one slip of the fingertip and you've told Dad rather than Dave.)

- **Reinvent the wheel** Strip for him? Puhleeze! You did that about a week into your sexual relationship, right? Now he's ready for the Blind Man's Strip. Blindfold him and sit him, fully clothed, on a chair in the middle of the room. Then proceed to strip for him while giving a running commentary on what you're up to. Dance and gyrate around and against him (letting leg, arms, breasts touch him briefly as you flaunt that flesh) and remove items of clothing. Stroke each item of clothing against his face, particularly under his nose, as it comes off, so that his other senses are stimulated. When you're completely stark naked, remove the blindfold but order him to keep his eyes shut until you say "open." When he does, it's to be treated to the sight of you, doing just that, sprawled on the bed, totally naked and totally ready for him.

Q: Why are more women having affairs?
A: Because they can

It used to be that women had affairs if they fell out of love with their husbands and in love with someone else. Then it became pseudo-acceptable (between friends, and as much as affairs are ever accepted) to have if-only-I-hadn't-drunk-so-much-I'd-never-have-done-it one-night slip-ups, if you weren't getting any at home. These days, a woman can be blissfully happy with her 2.5 children and white picket fence, be in love, and sexually satisfied by her husband – and still feel justified in having a bit on the side. Ask them why and they'll say "I deserve it," "It makes me feel alive." So who are these women, having two bites of the cherry? That girlfriend who travels for work. Women who work away from home (even if it's only twice a year) are twice as likely to have had two or more affairs during the past five years. The mother who's just waved off her last little one to preschool and for the first time in her life has time to herself. She decides to get her figure back and hubby, ironically, pays for the personal trainer as a present – who's 25, with the body of an Adonis and a Mrs. Robinson fixation. In fact, pretty well all surveys indicate that by the year 2010 the numbers of men and women having affairs will be equal, exploding the myth that the male is more adulterous by nature. Given half the chance, women cheat as much as men do. The only difference is that these days we've got just as many opportunities as he does. Interestingly though, while about 10 percent of men leave their long-term partners for their lovers, around one-third of women do. What remains true for both? The likelihood of an affair surviving as a long-term relationship is still slim. Possible moral of the story: if you're going to play men at their own game, play by their rules.

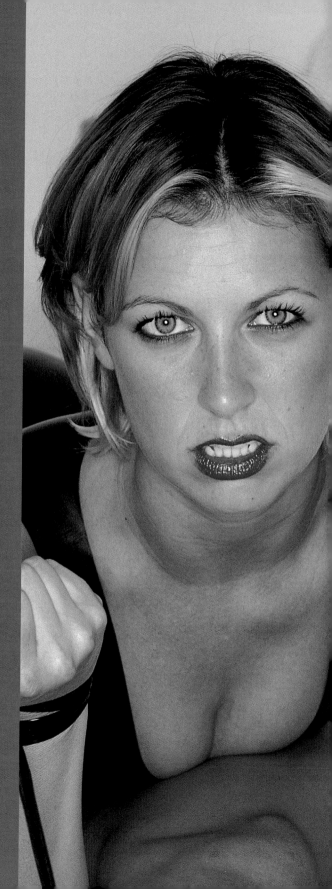

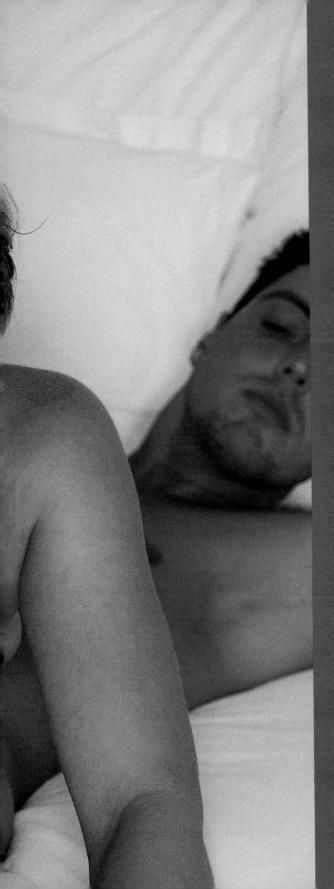

How many lovers is too many?

"Honey, ummm...I know this is none of my business. But..." Damn right it isn't! Confessing past lovers doesn't get you anywhere – except judged and possibly dumped. After all, isn't the definition of promiscuous simply someone who's slept with more people than you have? The short answer to "How many men have been here before me?": None of your business, darling. Here's why reducing your sexual history to a number doesn't work: I had three women over for coffee recently to be interviewed for a story. All were around 30. The first had slept with 26 men, the second four, and the third eight. No prizes for guessing which girl would be judged most harshly by a nosey boyfriend. But was she really the most promiscuous? Here's more information: The girl who's had 26 lovers has averaged around two lovers a year since she was 17 and been mainly single. The girl who'd slept with eight men put four notches in the bedpost during one weekend vacation sexfest while her then-husband stayed home and looked after the kids. The girl who slept with four had a threesome with two guys she met in a club. Outside, in an alley. She was 18 and a self-proclaimed wild child at the time. Now what do you think? I don't care who's asking – your boyfriend, mother, or the man at the local videostore – your answer to how many lovers you've had is no answer. (Only your gynecologist or the nice people at the clinic who are testing you for STDs have a right to know.) The reason you should keep your mouth zipped even if nothing else has happened, is that putting a number on your sexual history removes the emotion and circumstances. And don't kid yourself: if you blurt out a figure to your boyfriend, you'll be judged – and not necessarily by the same rules as he judges himself. Even if he's slept with 3,000, your three will be two too many.

Where did you learn that?
Perfecting your signature sex move

OK, I admit it: you're super, super close to supersexpert status if you've gotten this far (and you've done your homework). But to truly earn your great-in-bed badge, there's one thing you must perfect: a signature sex move. What's this exactly? Well, only you know the answer to that one. It might turn out to be a totally original complex maneuver, known only to you and your lovers. (You've not only patented it, but your exes know that if they so much as *think* of spilling your secret, you'll send in the heavies.) Or it could be something as ingeniously simple as a twirl of the tongue, done with such panache, it defies description (and so do you for doing it). Need some help to figure out your personal *pièce de résistance*? All it takes is a little thought and (perhaps) a lot of practice. Keep reading…

FOUR STEPS TO FINDING YOUR OWN SIGNATURE SEX MOVE

1. **Decide what you're best at**   The trick is to focus on whatever sex act you enjoy the most. If you like doing something, you're usually good at it – and if you're good at something, you usually enjoy it. So you can't really go wrong if you stick to this simple rule. If giving him a hand-job is your idea of hell, that's not going to be the area where you excel. If you could cheerfully massage him all day long, however, there's your starting point. Teach yourself some sensual massage techniques, top the whole delicious experience off with some erotic genital massage (see Hands On! pp.68–73, for inspiration and instructions) and there you have it: a mind-blowing move he won't forget in a hurry.

2. **Tap into your talent**   Decided on an area that you think holds promise? Try out a few different techniques before deciding on one to concentrate on. For the sake of this exercise, let's say that you've decided to become the absolute master/mistress of oral sex (I know, I am a woman obsessed). The next time you do it, ask your partner for a running commentary of how different techniques feel. Get them to rate each and every flick of the tongue on a scale of one to ten. What happens when you lick this part? What about that one? Now alter the pressure, carefully noting whether you're going up or down in the ratings game.

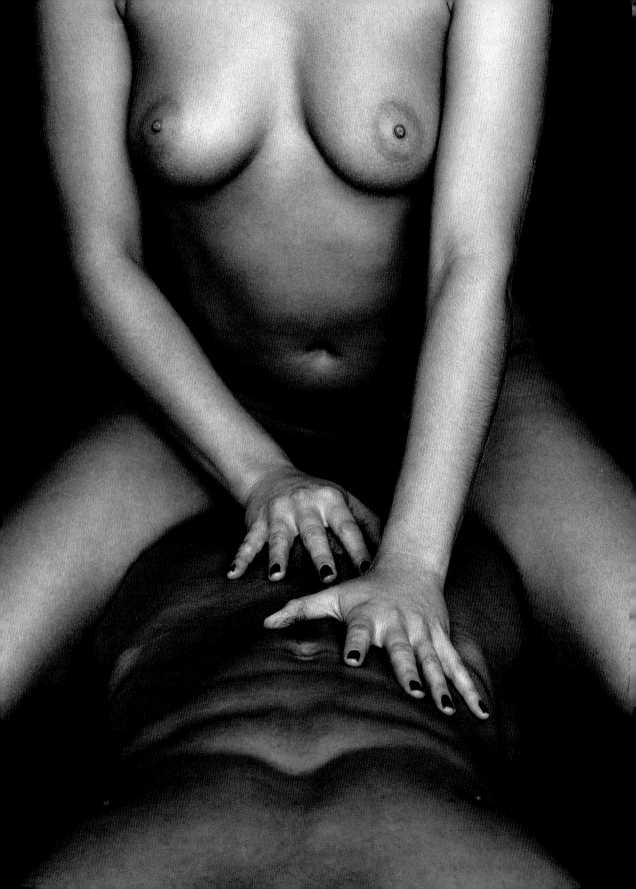

What happens if you add a twist of the wrist? Or start humming while you're doing it? Or refuse to break eye contact so that you see pleasure contort every feature of their face during orgasm? What about if you do the whole thing from start to finish in total and utter silence, like a slave? Or make so much noise, that they suspect you're enjoying the whole thing more than they are?

She has to **guess what's touching her now**, and every time she gets it wrong, **she gets the hairbrush again.** Weird how she's now **starting to like it…**

What about if you do the whole thing in slow motion? Speeded up? Or slicked up with lots of lubricant? Yes, it does take a few sessions to try it all out but then I can't see your partner complaining, can you?

3. **Ask around** Think you've found an erotic innovation that's uniquely yours? Do a quick survey of all your friends to find out how common it is and how well it's likely to be received. No need to confess what you're up to, just wait until everyone's had a few drinks and start a general conversation about it. Say you read a story that oral sex is the "Favorite Sex Act Of All Time." Do they agree? What makes it so great? What's the best oral they've ever had? Why? What do they think is the best tip they've ever done/heard of? Make sure you ask a mix of same- and opposite-sex friends to get both perspectives. If you're too embarrassed to ask face to face, do it via email. Say a friend of a friend is a magazine writer and is doing research for a story: you're helping them out by asking friends for hints and tips. Still convinced you've hit on something unusual enough to be noticed and appreciated? Round off your education by buying a good sex book that specializes in the area you've chosen. Or rent a sexy how-to-do-it film that illustrates it for you.

4. **Try it out!** Let all the hints, tricks, tips, and research merge into one spectacular sex session with your lucky, lucky, lucky partner. At first, concentrate hard on combining everything you've learned. Once you're in the swing, relax into it and let your gut instinct guide you. After all, you chose this because you LIKE doing it, remember? Sneak a peek to see how they're enjoying the sensation. Eyes rolled back in their head as they ecstatically orbit off the bed and the planet as well? Never mind, you'll do better next time. Tee-hee. Only one thing left to do now: give yourself a big pat on the back. Well, you can when you get your hands back.

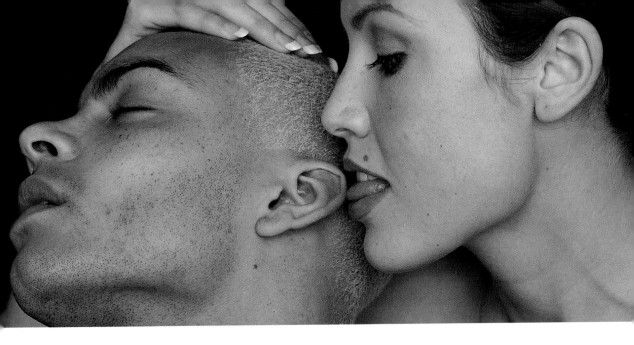

A LITTLE LOW ON INSPIRATION? THEN CLAIM ONE OF THESE AS YOUR OWN

- Pull on long, black satin gloves before you masturbate him. Use (unscented) talcum powder instead of lubricant; it's just as slippery (and comes out a lot easier in the wash).
- It's an oldie but a goodie, although everyone talks about it more than they actually do it. Break the mold: suck her toes and lick the spaces in between them.
- The no-hands massage. Start by straddling his back, then lean forward and use your breasts and upper body to massage his. From there, move into sliding your entire body length and genitals over his back, thighs, legs, and bottom (so you're climbing all over him and rubbing your body against him at the same time). The bonus with this one is that it feels just as good on your end as his.
- Blindfold her and get together a collection of everyday items with different textures – ones that feel nice against the skin and those that don't. Start with something that doesn't feel great – like a hard hairbrush – and swipe (but not too firmly) across her bottom. Then follow up with three or four items that produce good sensations. She has to guess what's touching her, and every time she gets it wrong, she gets the hairbrush again. Weird how she's now starting to like it…
- Look him straight in the eyes and talk very dirty. Simple but oh-so-effective.
- Buy a hand-held shower attachment. Get her to jump in, soap her up, rinse her off, then direct the flow right onto the clitoris. It won't be the first time she's enjoyed the sensuous feel of rushing water over her clitoris – why do you think women love spas so much? – but it will be the first time you've done it for her.
- Get him to pretend to be fast asleep. Then whisper the instructions so the game can commence: he must stay asleep to get the treats you've got in store for him. You then proceed to caress, lick, stroke, and suck every inch of his body, stopping the instant he "wakes" up. (If you start to hear real snores, you may need to up the activities a bit.)

7

SUPERSEXPERT

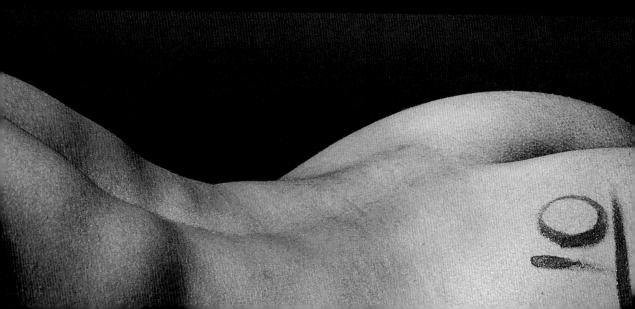

Do you really qualify as a supersexpert? Is your partner on their knees begging for **more, more, more**? Oh, all right then – here's your diploma. But only if you can check off the **eight things you should have done** in bed by now…

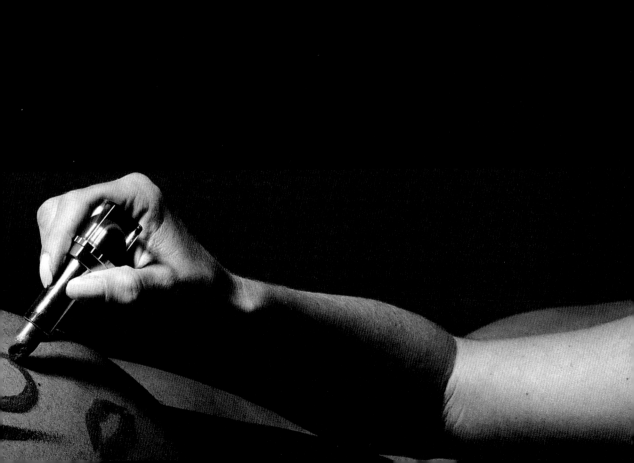

Graduation day
Making the grade at sex school

So you think you're ready to graduate from sex school? Good for you! As a supersexpert, you obviously know the 10 golden rules of fantastically great sex. Memorize all of them before you put on that mortarboard and clutch your diploma. (Better still: skip the ceremony and head straight for the party. Those hats never did anything for anyone.)

1. USE IT OR LOSE IT

Sex problems often aren't sex problems at all, they're time problems. If you have to hire in time management consultants to achieve this, do it: sort your life out so that you're making time for two sex sessions a week. I don't care if the grand total of time spent on these two sessions is 10 minutes. I just want you connecting sexually twice a week, minimum, unless you've got a really good reason not to (like you've just had a child). Ideally, you'll do it three times. If you really want to impress, it would be nice if you spent at least 10 minutes on two of those sessions and set aside 30–45 minutes for the final one. That's a commitment of around ONE HOUR for each week. Come on! I'm hardly asking for blood here.

Now, I know what a lot of you are thinking. That's nothing! She's undercalling it! Before you get too smug though, here's a few stats. A quarter of couples have sex once a week. A third have it twice. Only 15 percent have sex three times a week. Sixty-one percent say a long session lasts 45 minutes. Five percent of people watch TV while they're doing it. So this explains why I'm not being too ambitious. Time yourself. Most people don't spend as much time having sex as they think they do. There are lots of reasons why you should have regular sex. One big payoff: more orgasms, less effort. The more you have sex, the quicker the chemical connection between brain cells because the impulses are traveling along a well-beaten path.

2. BUY A VIBRATOR

Twenty-six percent of women in the US have used a vibrator at least once. Some drugstores stocked massagers for general aches and pains in the 1940s (does anyone know anyone who's actually used them to massage their shoulders? Exactly). Personally, I think the best vibrators are still those marketed as body massagers. They're less embarrassing to buy and all we need is a nice flat, small surface and good, strong vibration.

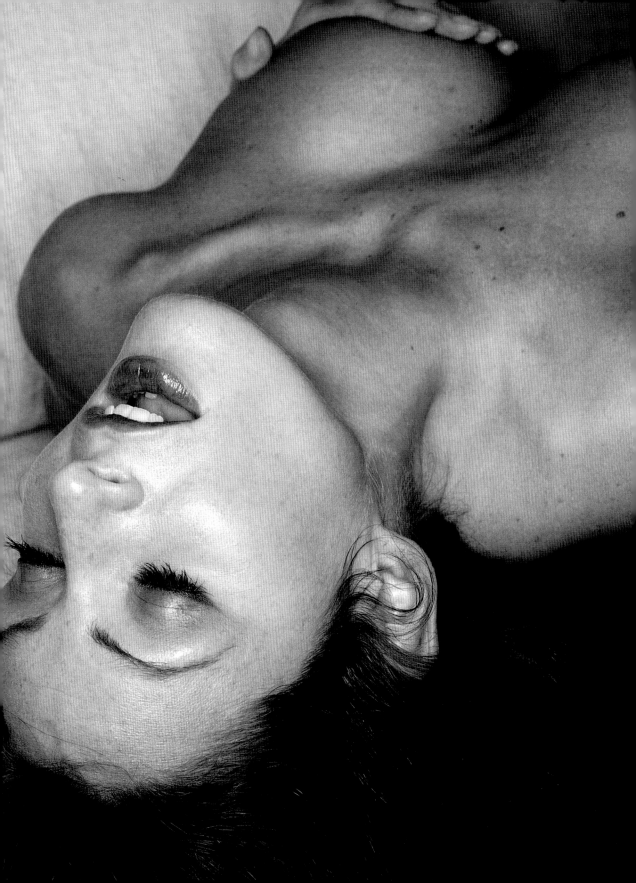

We don't need them phallic-shaped because most women don't insert them. Sorry guys. Yet another fantasy down the toilet! In fact, if ever you needed a perfect illustration of the way men see women's sexuality and how it really is, look no further than the humble vibrator. The versions designed by men: big, intense vibration (hence loud), and very phallic. Why he thinks it'll do the job: she'll obviously insert it and big is always best. The new versions, designed by women (who now have enormous sway in the sex aid industry with the rise and rise of women's erotic outlets): small, quiet, different speeds to suit different moods. If they're phallic-shaped, they've invariably got clitoral attachments. Or they don't resemble a penis at all. Instead, they masquerade as lipsticks, pebbles, rings…

If you're thinking **"who cares!"** you've got **the right attitude.** After all, you're having sex, not **performing live on TV.**

The world's favorite vibrator   The Rampant Rabbit – made famous by its guest appearance on TV show *Sex and the City*. It's got a bead-filled rotating shaft, a clitoral massager shaped like bunny-ears – and it sells more than one million a year.

New kid on the block   Make friends with Flipper the Dipper (or one of its many spin-offs), the couple-friendly vibrating device. It's a combination of a penis ring (designed to keep his erection hard by stopping the blood from escaping) and a vibrator. The jellylike ring fits over the base of his penis and has a built-in vibrating nub to stimulate your clitoris directly. The idea is to speed up your orgasm and slow down his. Sheer brilliance! Available from Ann Summers (www.annsummers.com). While you're on the net, have a browse through Good Vibes website (www.goodvibes.com); and for some extraordinarily beautiful sex aids, created by top designers (you seriously will want to leave them on the coffee table) check out www.myla.com. These really are future of sex gadgetry.

3. GO FOR CHEMISTRY

Think about the most mind-blowing sex you've ever had. Did you have the required 30 minutes of foreplay? Were you in the perfect position for intercourse where your clitoris could be stimulated? Hardly. Bet you both just ripped your clothes off and went for it. The ingredient responsible: chemistry. It's impossible to have take-my-house-car-children-cash-everything-just-give-it-to-me sex without it. While you do need all the technical stuff to keep it going long-term, finding your sexual soulmate makes the whole thing soooo much easier. If you've got colossal chemistry, everything else seems to click into place. The clothes come off and no one's embarrassed about their fat tummy or loony underwear; you're so caught up in the moment, you forget to worry about the silly stuff. You seem to hone in on each other's erogenous zones naturally (probably because you spend so much time in bed and explore everywhere). The only real problem about chemistry can be the person we've got it with. If they're forbidden, chemistry tends to move into overdrive rather than sensibly retreating. Instead of waving a white flag, if it hits the wrong target, it'll wave a note saying "Meet me in the broom closet at midnight." Which is often why the absolutely best sex you've ever had is with someone you shouldn't have been having it with. Hence why most people look guilty when asked the question "What's your most memorable sexual moment?" at a dinner party with close couple friends. (The correct response? Bat eyelashes at current partner and say "I never kiss and tell," while ignoring simultaneous kicks under table from your best friend who knows the truth.)

4. LAUGH IT OFF

Sex is smelly, noisy, sweaty, and unflattering. And if you've never done anything in bed that's caused you the slightest bit of embarrassment, you win the award for The World's Most Boring Lover. The World's Best Lover has had semen in their eye and pubic hair in their mouth, broken wind at the worst possible moment, looked down at their body and thought "God! I really should have joined that gym," tripped over because their panties were around their ankles, and woken up looking like a panda on Prozac (it's a girl thing, to do with smudged mascara and…oh, never mind). Anyway, if you're thinking, "who cares," you've got the right attitude. After all, you're having sex, not performing live on TV.

5. SEPARATE SEX FROM LOVE

Sorry to pour cold water on those romantic fantasies, but great sex and true love don't go together like bacon and eggs. Don't get me wrong, I'm with you: falling in love is one of life's most wonderful experiences. When it's reciprocated, it's like traveling on one big, fluffy white cloud: light, dreamy, and full of joy. When it's not, it's like being caught in the center of a vicious storm: you're battered, bruised, and bashed. Smart people figure this one out early on: just because your bodies fit, doesn't mean your hearts will too. Practice safe sex in all senses: don't have sex without a condom and don't wear your heart on your sleeve. Refuse to be treated badly. Choose partners who are confident people, happy in their own skins: the better they feel about themselves, the better they'll treat you.

6. STAY FAITHFUL

There's a problem with having a bit on the side. And listen, I'm not denying the appeal. If we're being totally honest (and the whole point of this book is to be just that), no one's denying that our libidos are revived spectacularly by a new playmate. The problem is, the excitement quickly fades and you're left with the same old problems again. It's the grass-is-greener syndrome. The sex feels great the first few times because of the newness and the "taboo" infidelity buzz, but once you're used to the new body and (even more of a passion killer) you're allowed to be with this person (the kiss of death for practically all affairs), boredom settles in. Unless you intend to spend the rest of your life skipping on to greener pastures, this is why working on making sex great with the same person is a really good idea.

7. SAY NO WITHOUT FEELING GUILTY

It's OK NOT to have – or even want – sex all the time. Forget the sitcoms, movies, and that boastful best friend: everyone's libido waxes and wanes, affected by hormones and stress levels, career demands, children, and health. If the only thing you want to do in bed right now is sleep, fine. Most partners would prefer that you said no instead of performing on demand begrudgingly. There's another reason why saying no occasionally could be a good idea: your sex life might actually be more exciting because of it. The odd refusal adds unpredictability. The minute sex becomes a foregone conclusion, you remove the thrill and chase from the relationship. Not the best idea you've had. How to say thanks but no thanks without offending? Instead of "Not tonight, Josephine," try "Let's wait until the weekend, so we don't have to rush and can really enjoy it."

8. MASTER THE CONDOM

What good is it when you're a committed couple? Well, you might want to use them for contraception rather than as just germ-catchers. And they're handy if you've got thrush or cystitis and don't want to play the let's-pass-it-back-and-forth game. For singles, they're a necessary evil but much less intrusive if you make them part of foreplay. Come on girls! Don't always leave it up to him to do the deed. It's far more exciting when it's your fingers unrolling it down the shaft (after squeezing air out of the tip first). If you can cope with the taste, he'll love it if you use your mouth to put on the condom. Hold it in position (the open end facing upward on your tongue). Cheat the first time and use your fingers to position it over the head of the penis, then use your tongue and mouth to unroll.

9. USE YOUR BRAIN

A true supersexpert has wised up to all
the myths and realized: 1. Your best
friend isn't getting it more than you are;
2. Simultaneous orgasms are rarer than hen's teeth;
3. Movie sex isn't even remotely close to the real thing;
and (the clinchers) 4. Real men have erection problems;
and 5. Real women have problems reaching orgasm. In fact,
plenty of women wish their sexual organs came not only with an
instruction manual, but with a lifetime warranty as well. Sometimes it would
be far simpler to send them back with a letter saying, "Send replacement. This one
only seems to work every third time," than it is to understand the sophisticated,
complicated workings of our clitoris. Why hasn't there been an *en masse* women's rally

The World's **Best Lover** has broken wind at the worst possible moment, tripped over because **their panties were around their ankles** and woken up **looking like a panda on Prozac.**

outside God's apartment? One reason might be answered by this statistic: How many orgasms is it
considered extraordinary to have in one session? Men: 4. Women: 6 to 50 (recorded by Masters
and Johnson in the US and the woman who put her hand up claimed she could have kept on
going if the researchers had not run out of men). Mind you, it obviously doesn't hurt to use your
brain and figure all this out. Forget the bimbette who's Babe of the Bedroom. If you want a girl
who really knows her stuff, choose the career girl. One survey found the two best predictors for
whether a woman could orgasm through sex were education and social status. Better-educated
women with higher professional status were much more likely to orgasm. Surely this settles the
"Which is better: bigger brain or bigger breasts?" argument once and for all.

10. OPEN YOUR EYES

Close your eyes on orgasm and you'll have an intensely pleasurable private experience. You
can focus properly on all the sensations flooding your body, play your favorite fantasy through
your mind, retreat into a wonderful world inhabited only by you, your body, your feelings, and your
orgasm. I agree — it's mind-blowing stuff. But if you really want to blast into Planet Supersex, keep
your eyes open. Look at your partner's face, watching the expressions that flit across it as they
experience pure pleasure, and suddenly orgasm becomes a shared experience. After all —
isn't that what it's all about?

GRADUATING GRACEFULLY

Now (drum roll), the final ingredient you need to be
a supersexpert! Is it a so-hot-it's-patented tongue technique?
An all-important hand maneuver? Prime position that guarantees
simultaneous orgasm each and every time? Nope. It's a hundred times more
important and effective than all of those combined. In fact, without it, virtually all the tips
and hints and how-to's in this book are rendered pretty useless. Come on, surely you've
guessed by now? It's sexual self-confidence — believing you're a sexy person, inside and out. Sort
of crucial, don't you think? That is why I want to have a final word about what's on the outside. I've
touched a little (if a lot of times) on how "sexy" comes from within and how what you feel like is
a lot more important than what you look like. I've also talked a little about genital appearance, and
size. What I've yet to address thoroughly, though, is what I think is a rather alarming trend toward
genital cosmetic surgery: the whole "designer vagina" and predilection to penis surgery thing.

If they're **forbidden, chemistry** tends to **move into overdrive** rather than sensibly retreating. Instead of waving the white flag, it'll wave a note sayir "Meet me in the **broom closet at midnight."**

My inclination is to ignore it in the hope that it will go away, but like everything else that
promises a quick, shortcut solution to a highly emotional issue, it's appealing — and dangerous.
Which is why I thought I'd give you the facts so that you can make up your own mind about it.
Tee-hee. (As if any of you would still plan to go ahead after reading all of this…)

THE SEAMLESS PENIS?

OK, I'm going to talk to guys first, so let's deal with some facts. Just in case you didn't pay attention in
"Penis Genius" (see pp.76–81): the average penis, not erect, is around 1.5 inches (3.9cm) in width
and 3.5 inches (9.5cm long). Erect, the average penis is around 5–7 inches (13–18cm) long — the
average is 6.2 inches (15.7cm) though some go up to 10 inches (26cm) — and about 5 inches
(13cm) in circumference — though some guys swell to 8 inches (20cm) and others are as small as
2.3 inches (6cm). And, by the way, if you're comparing yourself to the guy next to you at the urinal,
forget it. It's misleading to compare flaccid penises because the smallest nonerect penis can inflate
quite magnificently once erect, whereas a larger one might not change in size that much at all.
Anyway, that'll give you an idea of what's usual. As for what's considered small: a "micropenis" is what
the medical profession calls organs measuring as little as half an inch (1cm) erect. Since no exercise,
pill, cream, or vitamin will increase the size of your penis (and some will harm you: pump devices, for
instance, have been known to damage the fragile erectile tissue), it would be understandable, in this
case (and this case — micropenis — only), to consider penis enlargement surgery.

Here's how it works: contrary to popular belief, they don't usually add length during the operation but "release" length already there, coiled beneath the surface. The surgeon snips at the suspensory ligament that attaches the penis to the front of the pubic bone and *boing!* the extra length unfurls. It's the root of the penis, which is hidden in the pubic mound and can extend the penis by up to 50 percent of its original length. Be forewarned though, there is scarring, not to mention the usual risks of any surgery, along with possible loss of sensation. The most common technique designed to increase width of the penis involves sucking fat from the abdomen and injecting it under the penis skin. It's called CAPE (circumferential autolongous penile engorgement) and, if it's successful, fat cells attach themselves to the shaft and – presto! – your penis is wider. Hang on, though, before you go rushing out the door waving your credit card: the side-effects aren't pleasant if it's unsuccessful. The fat cells die, the fat deposits harden and the penis becomes, well, lumpy. Personally, I'd think long and hard (sorry) before taking the risk and ending up with a penis that looks like someone didn't stir the sauce properly. It's a pretty drastic, not to mention expensive, option.

Personally I'd think **long and hard** (sorry) before taking the risk and ending up with a penis that looks like **someone didn't stir the sauce** properly.

DESIGNER VAGINAS

As for getting a surgeon to operate on your vagina to make it look prettier – puhleeze! Personally, I think anyone who lets a surgeon come anywhere near the nerve endings of their clitoris, armed with a device that could potentially destroy them, is completely and utterly crazy. Women usually get their genitals operated on for two reasons: vaginal tightening or labia tidy-ups. Usually it's postbirth that women start to feel too "loose." Instead of doing kegel exercises, which would tighten things up nicely, some women take the surgery shortcut. This involves the vaginal wall muscles being stitched closer together to make the canal smaller. Some women ask to be "as tight as a virgin," while others want to be as they were before having kids, but basically you can order whatever size you want. Some women (the really nutty ones) get the operation done if their partner isn't terribly well-endowed so that sex is more "satisfying" for both of them. Labiaplasty is an operation where the doctor clips the outer sections of the labia to make them shorter or shapes the lips so they have a more symmetrical look. It's basically a labial facelift and it's as risky as the above-belt version. Or perhaps even riskier, because few surgeons are truly skilled in the procedure and there's the risk of permanent loss of sensation if too much skin is removed or ultrasensitivity if a nerve is exposed.

As I said, forget it. And if you're at the point where you're still considering it, you need to flip right back to the front of this book and start again, because you've missed the point!

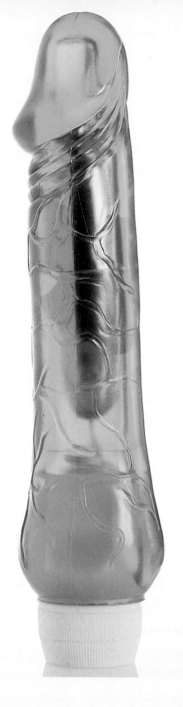

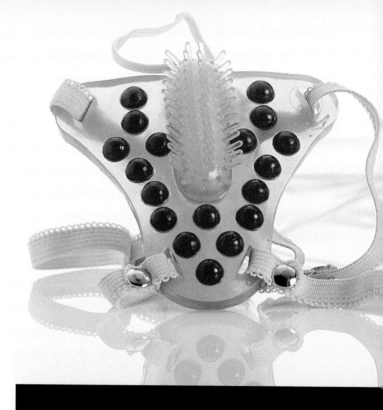

Sex toys

The first electric vibrators date back to Victorian times. When women were diagnosed as "neurotic" (they'd complain of a headache or cold) some doctors would administer an orgasm as treatment. Yes, really. Up went the skirts, down went the undies, and one white-coated arm disappeared upward to fumble around until the patient "released tension." It wasn't just Freud who thought that any and all female psychological/health/physical problems were related to sex: the medical profession heartily agreed. The vibrator was invented by a doctor who decided the whole "treatment" took too long when he used his fingers. A vibrator got the job done faster!

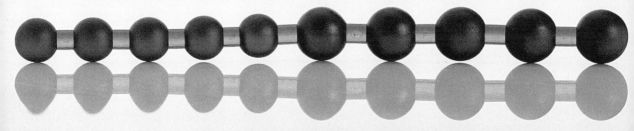

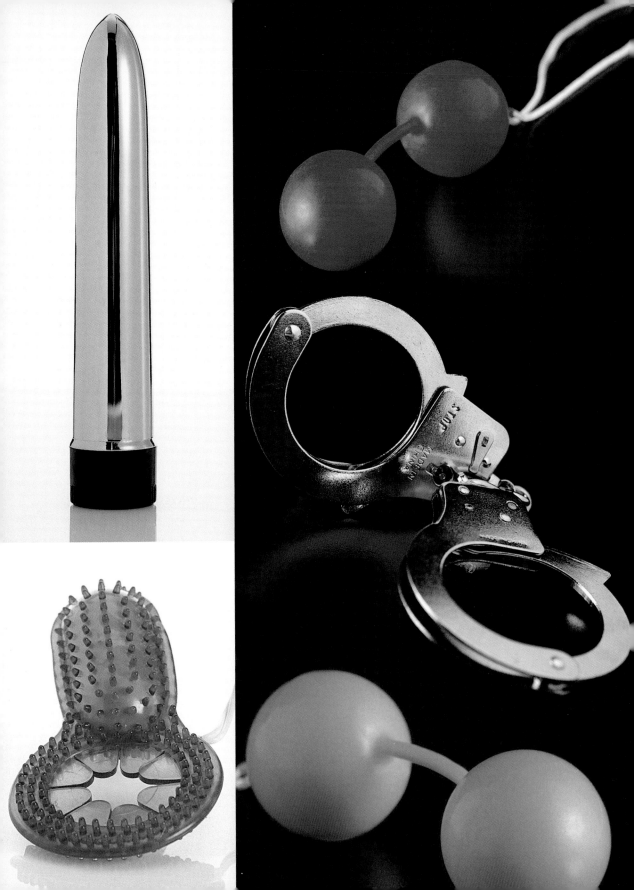

The best sex I ever had

Real couples reveal all

Most of us, sadly, are on first-name basis with so-so sex. Thankfully, for most this is also balanced by a fair smattering of great sex sessions. But what about exceptional sex? When you didn't just go to heaven, but were introduced to God and also got his autograph. What are the ingredients that make sex truly unforgettable? I asked a mix of people to look at a lifetime of intimacy and 'fess up to the naughtiest times. Here's a selection of their trips down most-memorable lane and the sexperiences they'll never forget. What made their finest sexual hour (or so) so special? Read carefully, you might just pick up a thing or two…

THE S-L-O-W TEASE

"I'd just come out of a really serious long-term relationship and met this guy at a boozy lunch at a friend's house. He was definitely not my type (not the sharpest knife in the drawer) but he had a body to die for and a great sense of humor. Over the next six weeks we hung around together and flirted like crazy, but I felt too raw emotionally to sleep with him. Instead, we'd kiss and touch (nothing heavy) and it turned into the most deliciously drawn-out sexual tease I've ever had. Toward the end, I was so turned on that all he had to do was kiss my neck and I'd practically orgasm! It was worth the wait: when I was finally ready, he led me into the bedroom and we didn't come out for 10 hours."

What made it great "It had all the essentials, which I call 'the three Ts': tease, talk, technique. The build-up was extraordinary, but it also helped that he was incredibly nonjudgmental and I felt comfortable talking to him about sex. He'd obviously been around the block a few times because he knew exactly what he was doing. Also, it was no-strings sex with an expiration date. The pressure of being Ms. Pure was lifted because I wasn't auditioning for the role of wife and I was able to let loose completely. Lack of emotional involvement meant I could just focus on the sex."

FLESH FOR FANTASY

"We'd fantasized lots of times about what it would be like for her to be nude on a stage, displaying herself for all to see – with me center stage, taking it all in and wanting to be up there, touching, feeling, licking, screwing. And then we did it for real. It's a strange feeling

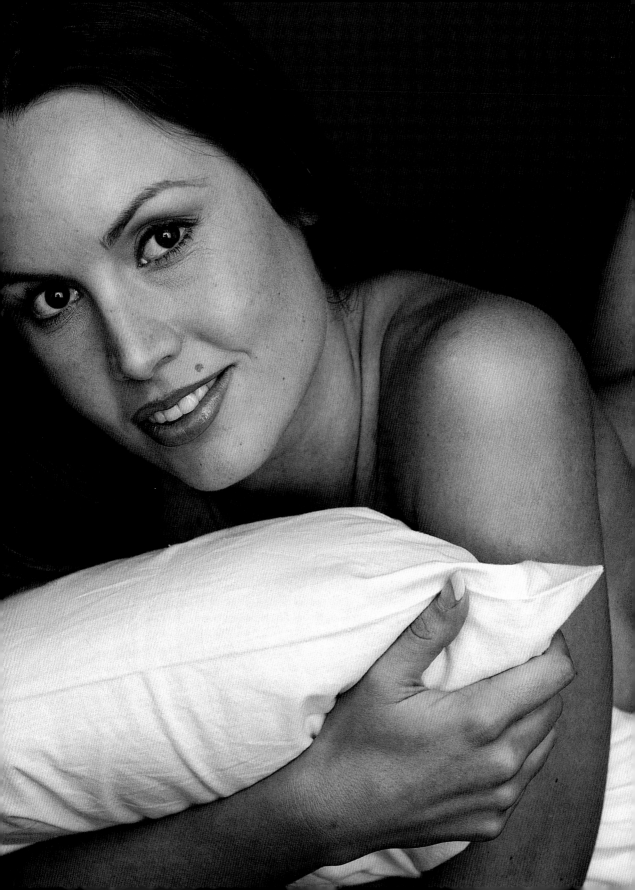

looking at your girlfriend – knowing exactly what she looks, feels, and tastes like, when she's in the company of a dozen other girls who you'll soon see buck naked on stage, all of them teasing the audience and trying to win the $100 prize. It was her idea to enter the competition but even so, I could tell she was as nervous as hell when it was her turn. But then she got into it and was just fantastic. I nearly came just by watching her. The finale was amazing: she laid back on the stage floor, spread her legs wide and ensured that every person in the room saw every inch of her nakedness. The sex when we got home was the best I've ever had and has still yet to be equaled."

What made it great   "The exhibitionism. All those guys looking at my girlfriend but knowing I was the only one who could sample the goodies. I also loved her sheer nerve – I don't think I could have done it!"

EX SEX

"My ex-boyfriend showed up to take me out. I wasn't sure whether it was now friendship or he was trying to get together again. But I did know I was as horny as hell. Anyway, all that stuff about pheromones must be true because after the briefest chat at the door, he made a joke about me looking good and wanting to ravish me, then said 'In fact, I will,' picked me up, and headed for the bedroom. We were both laughing when he threw me on the bed but then the mood changed. He started kissing and he told me (in graphic detail) exactly what he had wanted to do to me the last time we went out but was too scared to suggest. It's actually unlike him to indulge in dirty talk but I loved it! I asked him what he'd have liked me to do to him and he said to give him more blow-jobs. So I did. Then he asked me to masturbate for him and I did, while he watched, masturbating himself at the same time. We got up to all kinds of kinky stuff I'd never done before and – to be honest – haven't done since. Sadly."

What made it great   "We broke up because I thought he was a bit of a drip and too much in touch with his feminine side. I was always the one in control of the relationship, so him taking charge sexually, and quite forcefully, was a surprise. It blew me away! It was the role reversal combined with feeling safe enough to confess all these wicked fantasies that made it so hedonistic."

THE BEST OF THE REST...

For him

"Squeezing my testicles, just before orgasm."

"Watching her play with herself. She'd look me straight in the eye as she did it."

"She'd insert her finger up my butt while giving me oral sex."

"Giving me a blow-job while I was driving."

"Watching in mirrors above us, beside us, she had them placed everywhere."

"She used to bite my nipples hard, just as I was about to let go."

"Her tongue darting inside my anus."

"Her giving me head in a public place – the thrill of thinking we might be caught."

"She'd squirt lots of lube into her palms and rub them together, then masturbate me."

"Ordering me to climax in her mouth instead of trying to avoid it."

"Expecting to see pubes and then seeing her totally shaved genitals."

For her

"Being blindfolded and then feeling his tongue everywhere."

"Kissing another women while he watched."

"Realizing I had complete and utter control over him, physically and emotionally."

"The freedom to let loose and not caring if he judged me."

"Being the boss, ordering him around, treating him like a slave – like dirt, actually."

"Having a guy so fast after meeting him, I didn't even know his name – or want to find out."

"Talking dirty and saying all the stuff a woman's not supposed to."

"Giving in to lust, which didn't have a 'possible future relationship' tag on it."

"I can't decide which was better – the totally unexpected sexual encounter or the eagerly anticipated one that followed."

"Him making lots of noise while giving me oral."

"Lots of creative foreplay, gentle then rough, and I didn't ever want it to stop."

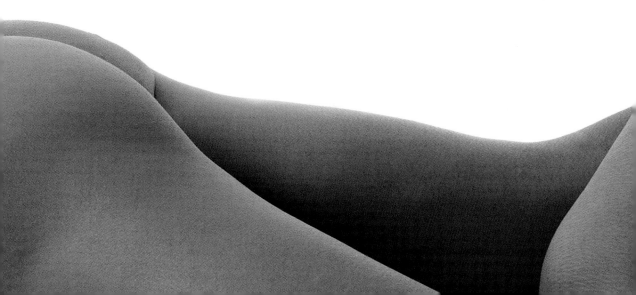

Index

Acknowledgments

The author would like to thank the following people:

Vicki McIvor, my extraordinary agent and special friend. This book wouldn't exist without you!

Everyone at DK, but most particularly Corinne Roberts, Deborah Wright, Christopher Davis, Bryn Walls, Mabel Chan, Stephanie Farrow, Serena Stent, and ultraspecial thanks to Peter Jones, who never once uttered the words "control freak," though God knows he must have thought it. DK stands for Dreadfully Kind. Also thanks to Daphne Razazan for initially welcoming me into the family.

Nigel and Bev from XAB for making the book look so fantastic, and John Davis for the stunning photographs.

And the following, for generously providing support (chocolate), information ("it only works if you put a pillow under your butt"), expertise ("if you ever tell anyone that story's about me, I will kill you"), practical tips ("you tickle right there and it's just amazing!"), and frank opinions ("penises aren't made of plasticine, you know"). Strangely, you all opted for being thrown into a group "thank," rather than singled out for your particular input. So here goes: Sandra Aldridge, Julian Aldridge, Jane Burniston, Neil Calow, Emma Dowson, Claire Faragher, Catherine and Ian Jarvie, Dan Genazzini, Pru McArthur, Lee Presland, and Alannah Richardson.

To all my friends for, again, putting up with me not being there for them when I should have been.

And to my family who might live far away, but couldn't be closer to my heart.

DK would like to thank Laurence Errington for the index.

The image used on pp.152–153 is from Photodisc.

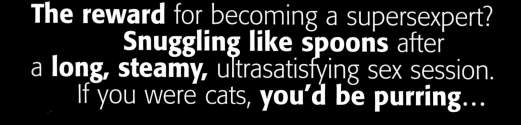

The reward for becoming a supersexpert?
Snuggling like spoons after
a **long, steamy,** ultrasatisfying sex session.
If you were cats, **you'd be purring**...

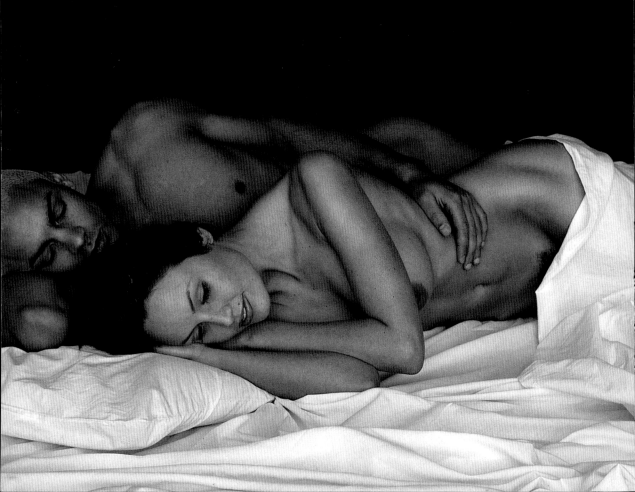